■ ■ ■

"Finally, a book with truth we can trust. Dr. Strand offers a priceless gift to improve the quality and quantity of life. Laser accurate and scientifically documented, it will help you win the war against degenerative disease and premature aging."

Denis Waitley, Ph.D., author
The Psychology of Winning

■ ■ ■

"At last, someone has written a book that explains, based on the medical literature, why we need to provide all the nutrients in supplementation to the cell in balance and at optimal levels. Everyone should read this book in order to begin taking control of their own health."

Dr. Myron Wentz,
Immunologist, microbiologist, and
founder of Gull Laboratories and USANA

■ ■ ■

This book is superbly written, and once I started reading it I could not put it down. I congratulate you on composing an excellent authoritative publication, which will be uselful for enlightening both physicians and patients alike on the health benefits of nutritional supplements.

M. Coyle Shea, M. D. F.A.C.S.

■ ■ ■

Thank you for your book, which I think is very well written and informative. I especially liked your comments regarding the label of "alternative medicine" as there is certainly nothing alternative about sound, rational, nutritional advice and supplementation to optimize the body's own defenses and healing potential.

Peter H. Langsjoen, M. D., F. A. C.C.

BIONUTRITION

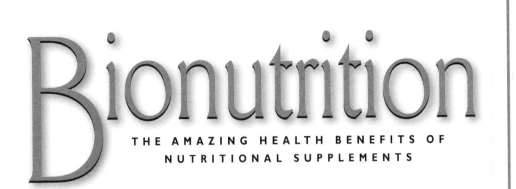

Bionutrition

THE AMAZING HEALTH BENEFITS OF NUTRITIONAL SUPPLEMENTS

Ray D. Strand, M.D.

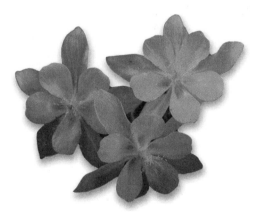

2ND EDITION

Comprehensive Wellness Publishing
Rapid City, SD 57709

For information, please contact
Comprehensive Wellness Publishing
P.O. Box 9226, Rapid City, SD 57709.

Every effort has been made to make this book as accurate as possible. The purpose of this book is to educate. It is a review of scientific evidence that is presented for information purposes. No individual should use the information in this book for self-diagnosis, treatment, or justification in accepting or declining any medical therapy for any health problems or diseases. Any application of the advice herein is at the reader's own discretion and risk. Therefore, any individual with a specific health problem or who is taking medications must first seek advice from their personal physician or health care provider before starting a nutrition program. The author and Comprehensive Wellness Publishing shall have neither liability nor responsibility to any person or entity with respect to loss, damage, or injury caused or alleged to be caused directly or indirectly by the information contained in this book. We assume no responsibility for errors, inaccuracies, omissions, or any inconsistency herein. Any slights of people, places, or organizations are unintentional.

First printing 1998
Second printing 1999

ISBN 0-9664075-7-1

LCCN 98-71598

Editing, design, typesetting and printing services provided by Sound Concepts, 500 South Geneva Road, Vineyard, Utah 84958 (Phone 801-225-9520). Cover Design and Art Direction by John M. Adams. ATTENTION MEDICAL FACILITIES, CORPORATIONS, UNIVERSITIES, COLLEGES, AND PROFESSIONAL ORGANIZATIONS: Quantity discounts are available on bulk purchases of this book for educational purposes. Special books or book excerpts can also be created to fit specific needs. For information, please contact Comprehensive Wellness Publishing, (888) 873-2590.

Table of Contents

Acknowledgments

I want to give a special thank you to Dr. Myron Wentz. His unwavering dedication in the fight against degenerative disease has truly been an inspiration. I also appreciate the boldness with which Dr. Kenneth Cooper is speaking out to the medical community in recommending that everyone needs to be taking nutritional supplements.

This book is a reality primarily because of my wife, Elizabeth. She has been a gift from the Lord. Her constant encouragement and loving support is what really kept my focus. With my busy private practice and strong commitment to my family, it was the late night hours that allowed me the time to complete the writing of this book. Thank you, Elizabeth, for continually reminding me I needed to finish what I had started. She has been a loving wife and a beautiful mother to my children: Donny, Nick, and Sarah. I am truly blessed.

The more I learn of how intricate our bodies are, the more I appreciate our divine design. This is not an accident. Our own bodies are our best defense against disease, especially when they are properly nourished. I must acknowledge His working in my life and His guidance in the writing of this book. We are marvelously and wonderfully made.

The Author

Introduction

Nothing curls physicians' toes more than when patients come into their office and ask if they should be taking nutritional supplements. I had all of the patented answers – they're snake oil; they just make expensive urine; one can get all the required nutrients by eating the right foods. If my patients persisted, I told them nutritional supplements probably wouldn't hurt them but they should take the cheapest they could find.

Maybe you have heard some of these same comments from your physician. For the first 23 years of my clinical practice, I simply did not believe in nutritional supplements. During the past five years, however, I have reconsidered my position based on recent studies published in the medical literature.

Should you be taking nutritional supplements? This book is dedicated to open-minded skeptics who are willing to look objectively at medical evidence. If you are a close-minded skeptic, you might as well put this book down now and save yourself a lot of time. Vitamins are an emotional issue within the medical field. One hopes logic will prevail and readers will begin to understand what is likely the next major breakthrough in medicine – nutritional science.

This book is dedicated to open-minded skeptics who are willing to look objectively at medical evidence.

Physicians are disease oriented. We look for disease. We are pharmaceutically trained to treat disease. We know our drugs. In medical school, we study pharmacology and learn how each of these drugs is absorbed, and when and how they are excreted from the body. We know the chemical pathways they disrupt to create a therapeutic effect. We learn their side-effect profile. We balance the therapeutic benefit of these drugs against their potential danger.

Pharmaceutical representatives try to gain access to our offices to display their goods. If that is not possible, they sponsor continuing medical education meetings in the hope of sharing their newest drugs. They highlight the latest double-blind, placebo-controlled clinical trial they believe supports the use of their drug in our patients. They take out full-page ads in national newspapers and magazines encouraging patients to talk to their physicians about their newest drug. You can't watch your favorite TV program without a pharmaceutical company selling its wares. This is the reality of medicine…This is the economics of medicine.

According to Peter Langsjoen, MD, a biochemist and cardiologist from Tyler, Texas:

> *Modern medicine seems to be based on an 'attack strategy,' a philosophy of treatment formed in response to the discovery of antibiotics and the development of surgical/anesthetic techniques. Disease is viewed as something that can be attacked selectively with antibiotics, chemotherapy, or surgery – assuming no harm to the host. Even chronic illnesses, such as diabetes and hypertension, yield simple numbers, which can be furiously assaulted with medications. Amidst the miracles and drama of the twentieth century we may have forgotten the importance of host support, as if time borrowed with medications and surgery were restorative in and of itself.*

He concludes by saying that disease-attacking strategies, along with host-supportive treatments, would yield much better results in clinical medicine.

The greatest defense against disease is our own body. Common sense tells us we need a strong and healthy immune system to protect our health. Nutritional supplements are needed to support the host (our bodies) in this battle against chronic disease. This is not in opposition to traditional medicine and all of our pharmaceutical and surgical advances. This is not alternative medicine. The main theme of this book is that supplements work along with pharmaceuticals and surgery to create significantly better results in clinical medicine.

Penicillin may help shorten the course of streptococcal throat infection by a few days. It also helps prevent rheumatic fever in younger patients. Without a strong immune system present within the patient, however, the treatment is of little value. A good example of this is infection in patients that are immunocompromised because of chemotherapy or complications from full-blown AIDS.

Most of the medical studies presented in this book are not from abstract medical journals. They are from main-line medical journals, such as the New England Journal of Medicine, Journal of the American Medical Association, The Lancet, and so forth. Pharmaceutical companies will not take out full-page ads to tell you about the health benefits of nutritional supplements. There isn't much money to be made by promoting natural products. Nutritional supplements cannot be patented via the Food and Drug Administration. It is up to physicians to take an open-minded look at these studies and be advocates for their patients.

I have been in the trenches of a private family practice for more than 26 years.

I have seen my share of gimmicks and quackery peddled to my patients. Physicians must be skeptical and protect their patients against any scheme or product that could be harmful to their health. Double-blind, placebo-controlled, clinical trials (the standard in clinical medicine) are needed to assess what truly benefits our patients and what does not. This is the type of evidence I present in this book.

In this age of biochemical research, where we are now able to determine what is happening in every part of each cell, the very essence of degenerative diseases is now coming to light. Oxygen necessary to sustain life on this planet also has a "dark side"– oxidative stress. One must understand how this affects the body and how to protect against it. This book is the culmination of three years of research into oxidative stress and how it relates to health and disease.

Prevention of disease is the first order of business for any physician. In the early 1970s, I began to recommend moderate exercise. Evidence in the medical literature now shows there is a health benefit with moderate exercise. In the 1980s, I recommended that my patients eat a low-fat, high-fiber diet with at least five to seven servings of fruits and vegetables each day. The medical literature convinced me there was a definite health benefit in this recommendation. Today I recommend nutritional supplements to my patients, which I am convinced offer definite health benefits to my patients. Therefore, my patients need to have a modest exercise program, eat a low-fat, high-fiber diet, and take high quality nutritional supplements in order to best protect their health. I firmly believe the medical literature strongly supports ALL of these recommendations. This is not alternative medicine – it is common sense preventive medicine.

When we provide the body with micronutrients at optimal levels, the body is able to function at a much higher level. Recommended Dietary Allowances (RDA) were developed to prevent acute nutritional deficiencies (scurvy, rickets, and pellagra). Bionutrition provides the optimal level of nutrients to prevent, or at least delay, chronic degenerative diseases (heart attack, stroke, and cancer) and to enable the body to do what God intended. Physicians across the country are now beginning to discover this truth. I sincerely hope this book benefits your health and your life.

SECTION I

One

Degenerative Disease
and Oxidative Stress

The twenty-first century is upon us and physicians and medical researchers are taking note of the status of health care in the world. In 1900, people died primarily of infectious diseases, such as pneumonia, tuberculosis, diphtheria, and influenza. Thanks to great advances in the development of antibiotics during the last half of the century, however, deaths caused by infectious diseases have declined dramatically. Now, the leading causes of death and disability are related to degenerative diseases, such as coronary artery disease, stroke, cancer, Alzheimer's dementia, arthritis, cataracts, macular degeneration, and so forth. Biomedical research has made great advances in the past decade in helping us understand the root cause of degenerative disease – oxidative stress. This book will explore these scientific advances and show how you can apply these principles to better protect your own health.

Millions of people around the world (including more than 60 million Americans suffer from some form of cardiovascular disease (disease of the heart and blood vessels). In the United States, where I live and practice medicine, 13,670,000 have coronary artery disease. Although there has been a significant decrease in the number of cardiovascular deaths in the past 25 years, cardiovascular disease still remains the number one cause of death in the United States and the industrialized world. There are 1.5 million heart attacks each year and about one-third of these heart attacks are fatal. Forty-five percent of these heart attacks occur in patients under the age of 65. The sad statistic is 250,000 of these deaths occur within the first hour of a heart attack, which does not even allow the patient enough time to make it to the hospital. Physicians realize that the first sign of heart disease in more than 30 percent of cases is sudden death. Therefore, prevention of heart disease takes on extreme importance. There is not much time for lifestyle changes in this group of heart patients.

In spite of the tremendous amount of money spent on cancer research and treatment, cancer remains the second leading cause of death in the United States. There were 537,000 cancer deaths in 1995 and 1.3 million new cases projected to be diagnosed in 1996. Unlike heart disease, there has been a steady increase in the number of deaths caused by cancer over the past 30 years. We have spent over $22 billion in cancer research over the past 25 years, only to see absolutely no decrease in the relative number of people dying from this disease. The greatest advancements in cancer treatment have developed because of earlier diagnoses of certain cancers. Everyone agrees we need to be looking more at primary prevention of cancer, since our treatments of cancer are very harsh and usually not very effective.

In 1950, the United States ranked seventh among the top 21 industrialized nations in the world when it came to life expectancy. Since that time, the U.S. has spent far more money on health care than any other country in the world. Last year it spent over $1 trillion on health care, which was 13.6 percent of its gross national product (GNP). That is well over twice as much as the next closest nation. We have our MRI and CT scanners, angioplasty, bypass surgery, total hip and knee replacement, chemotherapy, radiation therapy, antibiotics, advanced surgical techniques, advanced drugs, intensive care units – the list goes on and on.

In 1990, the U.S. ranked eighteenth in life expectancy compared to those same 21 industrialized nations. The healthcare system that Americans claim is the best in the world is actually near the worst when we look at how long Americans live.

We aren't getting our money's worth, especially when you consider how much we are suffering from the effects of chronic degenerative diseases. Look at the near-epidemic increase of Alzheimer's dementia, diabetes mellitus, arthritis, chronic obstructive lung disease (emphysema), and macular degeneration.

It is not the years of life with which most of us are concerned but the quality of life in those years.

It is not the years of life with which most of us are concerned but the quality of life in those years. Who would want to live to a ripe old age if you cannot recognize your closest family members because of Alzheimer's dementia? Or if you were unable to move without significant pain because of rheumatoid arthritis? Or if you lose your eyesight because of age-related macular degeneration? No one seems to die of old age any more. We are suffering and dying instead from chronic degenerative diseases.

We need to look again at our approach to health care. The overwhelming majority of our health care dollars are spent after we become sick. Little is spent on prevention. Our philosophy in medicine is to "attack" disease. Perhaps this came with the advent of antibiotics. With the vast array of medications to choose from one would think we could cure everything. We have not met with much success, however, when it comes to treating chronic degenerative diseases. At best we may be able to slow the process down, but usually we are simply just making patients more comfortable. Physicians must admit that our treatments for stroke, cancer, macular degeneration, Alzheimer's dementia, and Parkinson's disease are really not very effective.

As mentioned earlier, life itself is totally dependent upon oxygen, but there is a "dark side" of oxygen. There are now more than 50 chronic degenerative diseases that medical research scientists have shown to have oxidative stress as a major component. We are more or less "rusting" inside. This is the same process that causes iron to rust or a cut apple to turn brown. (This will be explained in greater detail in Chapter 2.) By understanding what causes oxidative stress and how we are best able to prevent its devastating effects in our bodies, we can learn how to decrease the risk of heart disease, stroke, cancer, Alzheimer's dementia, macular degeneration, arthritis, emphysema, and a host of other chronic degenerative diseases.

Prevention of chronic degenerative disease and protection of our health is the key. It is much easier to maintain your health than it is to regain it after it has been lost. Physicians must again learn to appreciate the fact that the host (our body) is the greatest defense against chronic degenerative diseases. Bionutrition is the best way to build up our body's natural antioxidant defense system as well as our own immune system. You will learn as you read this book that the best defense against chronic degenerative diseases is our own bodies – not the drugs that I prescribe in my office. Patients must become more proactive with their health if they are going to have any chance to protect themselves against these chronic degenerative diseases. You need to know about Winning the War Within if you want to have the best chance of maintaining your health.

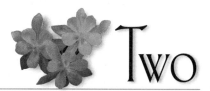

Two

The War Within

There is an oxygen "paradox": we cannot live without oxygen, yet it is
inherently dangerous to our existence. A war is being waged within every
cell of your body. It is called oxidative stress and is now believed to be a major
component in the development of more than 50 chronic degenerative diseases.[1]
The same process that causes iron to rust, cut apples to turn brown, or food to
decay is waging an out-and-out attack on every living cell in your body. We are
essentially rusting inside and are not even aware it is happening. We all must
gain understanding of this process and learn how to protect ourselves against its
terrible destruction.

THE ENEMY: FREE RADICALS

Free radicals are mainly oxygen molecules or atoms that have at least one
unpaired electron in their outer orbit. In the process of utilizing oxygen during
normal metabolism within the cell to create energy (called oxidation), active free
oxygen radicals are created. They essentially have an electrical charge and desire

to try to get an electron from any molecule or substance in the vicinity. They have such violent movement that they have been shown chemically to create bursts of light within the body. If these free radicals are not rapidly neutralized by an antioxidant, they may create even more volatile free radicals or cause damage to the vessel wall, cell membrane, lipids, proteins, and even the nucleus (DNA) of the cell. Our bodies are literally under attack.[2]

Imagine you are sitting in your living room on a cold night and a warm, beautiful, wood fire is burning in your fireplace. The fire burns safely most of the time. However, occasionally there is a "pop" and a cinder shoots out and lands on your carpet, burning a little hole in it. Now that isn't really a big deal. However, if this were allowed to continue month after month and year after year, you would have a pretty ragged carpet in front of your fireplace.

This is a great illustration of what is essentially happening inside our bodies. The sparks that shoot out of the fireplace are free radicals, and the tattered carpet is degenerative disease. Whatever part of the body wears out first determines what type of degenerative disease you will develop. Some research scientists even believe certain areas of our body are genetically predisposed to oxidative stress, which may explain familial traits when it comes to degenerative diseases.

THE ALLY: ANTIOXIDANTS

We are not totally defenseless against the attack of free radicals. We have our own army warring against the dark side of oxygen; they are called antioxidants. Antioxidants have the ability to render these free radicals harmless. Antioxidants are like those glass doors or the fine wire mesh we put in front of our fireplace. The sparks will continue to fly, but now they are contained and not allowed to injure or damage the carpet (our body). As long as there are adequate amounts of antioxidants within our bodies to handle the free radicals produced within the cell, there is no damage to the surrounding tissues.

The body has the ability to make some of its own antioxidants. Three major antioxidant systems that the body makes are superoxide dismutase (SOD), catalase, and glutathione peroxidase. However, the body is never able to produce enough antioxidants on its own to neutralize all of the free radicals that our bodies produce. We must get the rest of the antioxidants that we need from our food. If there are more free radicals produced than there are antioxidants available, oxidative stress occurs. If this situation is allowed to persist for any length of time, a chronic degenerative disease may develop. This is the war within.

Balance is the key to winning this war. There must always be an abundant supply of antioxidants within every cell and surrounding tissue to protect the body against the damage that can be caused by these free radicals. Beta-carotene, vitamin C, and vitamin E are the best known antioxidants. Vitamin C is a water-soluble vitamin and the most effective antioxidant within the blood and lung tissue; it also regenerates vitamin E. Vitamin E is a fat-soluble vitamin and is absolutely the most effective antioxidant within the cell membrane.

In addition to these vitamins, there are thousands of different antioxidants that we obtain from our foods, which are primarily found in our fruits and vegetables. They all work in synergistic fashion within our bodies, and the more that we have and the more varied they are, the better. Glutathione is one of the most potent antioxidants within the cell and works alongside superoxide dismutase. Alpha lipoic acid, mixed carotenoids, Coenzyme Q10, cruciferous, N-acetyl L-cysteine, lutein, and a host of bioflavonoids are examples of more antioxidants we are able to get from our foods. Not only do these antioxidants work in synergy with one another, but they also work against different types of free radicals in different parts of the body. They represent true teamwork because they are all needed if we are to have any chance of winning the war within.[3]

BEHIND THE LINES

There is a support system behind the battle lines which is critical in the struggle to win this war. Antioxidants by themselves are not the complete answer. They need adequate amounts of the so-called antioxidant minerals – copper, zinc, manganese, and selenium. There must also be adequate amounts of folic acid and vitamins B1, B2, B6, and B12, which are cofactors for the antioxidants. These nutrients are essential in the enzymatic reactions of the antioxidants so they are able to do their job on the front lines against the free radicals. In other words, if these minerals and cofactors are not present in adequate amounts, it decreases the effectiveness of the antioxidants that may be present. Oxidative stress may still occur. It is critical to remember: If the battle is going to be won, all these nutrients must be present in adequate amounts.

Although free-radical production occurs during normal metabolism, the amount of free radicals that the body produces is not static or steady. There are many factors that can significantly increase the amount of free radicals that our bodies produce.[4]

BIONUTRITION

EXCESSIVE EXERCISE

In his book The Antioxidant Revolution, Kenneth Cooper, MD, emphasizes that excessive exercise is a major cause of oxidative stress.[5] He became very concerned when he began seeing several of the super exercisers who had been coming to his aerobic center in Dallas dying from heart disease and cancer at an early age. He began researching the medical literature and started to realize that excessive exercise could actually be dangerous to our health. When we exercise mildly or moderately, the production of free radicals increases, but not significantly. When we exercise excessively, however, the production of free radicals goes off the graph, or in other words it increases exponentially. Dr. Cooper started the exercise craze back in the early 70's when he coined the term aerobics. He has never recommended excessive exercise to his patients; however, he had previously not discouraged it either. Now he believes it is potentially harmful to your health and should only be done by the serious, competitive athlete who is taking large amounts of antioxidants in supplementation. I agree. Dr. Cooper is now recommending a modest-to-moderate exercise program for his patients. He also informs them that they should be taking adequate levels of antioxidants in supplementation all the time. On the day that they exercise, he feels they should actually increase the amount of antioxidants they are taking.

EXCESSIVE STRESS

Just like exercise, we seem to be able to handle the modest increase in free-radical production found present with mild-to-moderate emotional stress. If we are under severe emotional stress, however, free-radical production again goes up exponentially and can cause significant oxidative stress. How many times have you known a close friend or family member who has been under tremendous stress for a prolonged period of time who developed their first heart attack or serious illness? Have you ever noticed that when you become exhausted, it is usually when you become very sick? I don't have many patients that have run 30 to 40 marathons in their lifetime; however, I have many patients who are under tremendous stress. Our lives have become so complicated by financial, work, and personal pressures. I believe that stress is the most important health factor that I deal with in my practice. Once you begin to understand oxidative stress and how emotional stress is one of the main triggers for producing free radicals, you begin to understand why it is so dangerous to our health.

POLLUTANTS IN OUR AIR, FOOD, AND WATER

People today are exposed to more chemicals and pollutants in our air, food, and water than ever before. Drive into any major city and you can literally taste the air. The Environmental Protection Agency states there are well over 70,000 chemicals being used commercially in the United States. New commercial chemicals are being produced at a rate of about 1,000 per year. Many of these are used in the production of our food; many end up in our water supply. In 1988 the U.S. Department of Public Health warned that 85 percent of U.S. drinking water was contaminated.

All of these chemicals and pollutants that enter our body must be handled in some way. Some are metabolized and excreted. Some toxins are stored, especially in our fat. However, all of these toxins significantly increase the amount of free radicals that the body produces. This generation is exposed to more oxidative stress caused by our environment than any previous generation in the history of the world. We have to live in this world. Therefore, we need to learn how to avoid as many pollutants and chemicals as possible and, at the same time, optimize our body's natural antioxidant defense system.

One of the greatest causes of oxidative stress is smoke from cigars and cigarettes.

CIGARETTE SMOKE

One of the greatest causes of oxidative stress is smoke from cigars and cigarettes. We all know that smoking is probably the greatest risk to our health. Many clinical studies have shown that cigarette smoke causes tremendous production of excess free radicals. There is also significant production of free radicals associated with secondary smoke. Laws are being passed every day to protect the public against being exposed to secondary smoke, and there is very solid clinical evidence that this is a risk factor to our health.

Antioxidants have been shown to decrease the oxidative stress in smokers. However, there is no way to eliminate its devastating effect on the body other than to quit. Many of my patients desire to quit smoking; however, nicotine is absolutely the most addictive drug with which I have to deal. The greatest thing that a smoker can do for his or her health is to quit. Those individuals who are able to quit smoking will not only add years to their lives but also quality to those years. The main reason that this is true is because you have just eliminated one of the main causes of oxidative stress for you and your family.

SUNLIGHT

Sunlight has been shown to greatly increase free-radical production within the skin. We have all been fooled into a false sense of security by the use of sunscreens. The irony of most sunscreens is the fact that they protect you from the sun's burning rays but not very well against the skin-damaging rays. Consequently, we actually spend more time out in the sun because we are not getting burned, but we are greatly increasing our risk of skin cancer. Make sure the sunscreen you use specifically states it offers adequate protection against both UVA and UVB sunlight. Clinical studies are proving that the mechanism of damage from the sun to our skin is via oxidative stress.

MEDICATIONS AND RADIATION

Medications are synthetic and are a foreign chemical to the body. The body must eliminate them. In this process it produces excess free radicals. Some of the greatest offenders are chemotherapeutic agents. Several studies show that many toxic effects to the body from chemotherapeutic drugs are a result of the oxidative stress they produce.

Radiation treatment causes tremendous increase in free-radical production and ultimately leads to oxidative stress, no matter what part of the body is exposed to the radiation. Obviously, plain x-rays and CT scans produce increased amounts of free radicals but not to the same extent as radiation therapy.

FATTY MEALS

A hamburger is not only going to elevate your cholesterol but has recently been shown to significantly increase the number of free radicals. This has been shown to actually damage the lining of, and may even cause spasms of, your arteries. When individuals take high doses of antioxidants with these fatty meals, these effects are eliminated.

THE BATTLE CONTINUES

Decreasing our exposure to these risk factors is a start, although it is impossible to eliminate all of them. We must live in our environment. Therefore, it is critical to our health to learn how we can optimize our antioxidant defense system to handle ever-changing levels of oxidative stress. Balance is the key to winning the war within. We must have enough antioxidants and their supporting nutrients available to handle all of the free radicals produced, or we will lose the battle. If oxidative stress is allowed to persist for a prolonged period of time, we will lose the war. This, then, is the very foundation for the mechanism of degenerative disease. In the coming chapters, you will begin to see oxidative stress is the common denominator of degenerative disease.

As we look at the overwhelming evidence in the medical literature in the following chapters, I believe you will become just as convinced as I am that nutritional supplementation is not only wise but essential in protecting our health. Evaluate the evidence with an open-minded skepticism.

In every battle, whether we win, lose, or draw, there are going to be casualties. Free radicals are going to inflict some damage on our cells, even if we have adequate antioxidants. However, the body has a great ability to heal itself. If we provide the nutritional building blocks to accomplish this repair, we can handle this assault on our cells. In health and disease, physicians must learn to respect the body's own ability to defend itself against oxidative stress and to repair this damage. I call this bionutrition. Simply defined, bionutrition means providing these essential micronutrients to the body at a level that has been shown in the medical literature to provide a health benefit.[1]

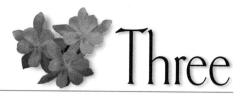

Three

Oxidized LDL Cholesterol
The Truly Bad Cholesterol

THE CHOLESTEROL STORY

When I began private practice in 1972, we did not pay much attention to cholesterol. We did measure total cholesterol, but the normal range listed on the chemistry panel at that time was 140 to 320. I told many patients who had a cholesterol level of 280 to 300 not to be concerned because this was well within the range of normal. By the mid-1970s, however, we began to argue the possibility that elevated cholesterol was an independent risk factor for heart disease. By 1980 there was overwhelming evidence in the medical literature that cholesterol was an independent risk factor for coronary artery disease.

The Framingham studies led the way for developing a new range of normal for cholesterol: 120 to 200. Individuals who maintained a cholesterol level of less than 150 did not develop coronary artery disease. As levels went up from there,

there was almost a straight-line increase in the risk of heart disease. Patients who had cholesterol between 150 and 200 had a low risk of developing coronary artery disease, those who had cholesterol between 200 and 240 were at moderate risk, and those with a cholesterol level above 240 were at high risk of developing coronary artery disease.

In the mid-1980s, studies showed us that not all cholesterol was bad. Low-density lipoprotein (LDL) was the bad cholesterol and high-density lipoprotein (HDL) was the good cholesterol. The higher the HDL cholesterol, the better. We actually developed a ratio between the total cholesterol and the good cholesterol. This has been a very important ratio for helping us to determine the overall risk of coronary artery disease in our patients. However, the LDL cholesterol was actually the bad cholesterol that built up in our arteries and helped to develop the plaque which is characteristic of hardening of the arteries. The HDL cholesterol actually cleans the LDL cholesterol from our vessels. The medical literature has now shown us to not only check a patient's total cholesterol but also to break it down into HDL and LDL cholesterol fractions. The higher the HDL (good) cholesterol, the lower your risk for developing coronary artery disease. The higher the LDL (bad) cholesterol, the higher the risk of developing coronary artery disease.

OXIDIZED LDL

Most readers probably have a good knowledge of the information shared here about cholesterol. But few have heard or truly understand the significance of the oxidized or modified LDL. Daniel Steinberg, MD, reported his theory of oxidized LDL in the April 6, 1989, issue of the New England Journal of Medicine.[1] He hypothesized that native LDL was not the culprit in the process of atherosclerosis (hardening of the arteries), but it needed to be oxidized by excess free radicals before it became "bad" cholesterol. This oxidation process usually took place in the intima, or lining of the vessel. Therefore, if the native LDL was able to resist this oxidation process, the bad cholesterol was no longer bad. He theorized that if the LDL particle itself and the surrounding tissue contained enough antioxidants to prevent LDL cholesterol from oxidizing, the process of atherosclerosis could be significantly inhibited. Thus, the prevalence of cardiovascular

...cardiovascular disease in this country could possibly be reduced if people simply ate better and took nutritional supplements.

disease in this country could possibly be reduced if people simply ate better and took nutritional supplements.

Let's examine this medical research more closely. Oxidized or modified LDL is the type of cholesterol found in the plaque in arteries and is the basic component of hardening of the arteries. But how does it get there? Native LDL cholesterol is not the problem. If it becomes modified by excessive free radicals, however, oxidized LDL becomes dangerous.[2]

The process of hardening of the arteries begins as follows:

1. Coronary artery disease is now felt to be an inflammatory disease. Free radicals, oxidized LDL, homocysteine, infectious agents, hypertension, and even fatty meals irritate the surface lining of the artery called the intima or endothelium. This causes either a disruption or dysfunction of the intima.

2. Oxidized LDL is then allowed to get into the lining of the artery through this disruption or dysfunction of the endothelium. It is actually acting as a Band-Aid in an attempt to try to heal this injury to the lining of the vessel wall.

3. Oxidized LDL attracts a white cell called a monocyte.

4. The monocyte changes into a macrophage, which is like the video game Pac-Man. This macrophage then begins to gobble up the oxidized LDL until it is totally stuffed. This creates a foam cell, which look just like you would imagine.

5. Foam cells become loaded with this oxidized LDL fat.

6. Foam cells attach to the vessel wall and begin to form a fatty streak. This is the first sign of hardening of the arteries – and it all started with the inflammation of the lining of the artery. This allowed entry of the oxidized LDL into the surface just under the lining of the artery.

Thus, the link between the oxidation of the LDL cholesterol and atherogenesis (hardening of the arteries) provides a simple rationale for the beneficial effect of antioxidants on the incidence of coronary artery disease. Since Dr. Steinberg's article appeared in 1989, there have been several epidemiological studies and clinical trials relating the use of antioxidants in altering the course of atherosclerosis.

RELATION OF RESISTANCE TO OXIDATION OF THE
LDL CHOLESTEROL AND ATHEROSCLEROSIS

There have been numerous studies in animals and in humans that have shown that the higher the level of antioxidants within the LDL cholesterol and the surrounding cells, the more resistant the LDL cholesterol is to the oxidation process.[3,4,5] Vitamin E (a fat-soluble vitamin) has been the most extensively studied antioxidant. It is actually incorporated into the LDL particle itself. This is of great importance since wherever the LDL cholesterol goes, so will the vitamin E. There is strong clinical evidence that demonstrates where there are adequate antioxidants in the LDL particle and surrounding cells, oxidative modification of the LDL does not occur. By supplementing the plasma with vitamin E, researchers were able to demonstrate increases in the level of vitamin E in the LDL cholesterol itself. They demonstrated that the higher the vitamin E content of the LDL cholesterol, the higher the resistance was of the LDL to oxidative modification. This appeared to be nearly a linear response, that is, the higher the vitamin E level the greater the resistance. Vitamin E is a very important antioxidant but definitely not the only antioxidant needed to help protect the LDL.

Mixed carotenoids have also been shown to provide protection to LDL cholesterol.[6] Vitamin C offers the best protection to LDL cholesterol within the plasma. Intracellular antioxidants, such as glutathione and N-acetyl L-cysteine, are also very important. Cellular antioxidant activity is critical in maintaining the balance of free radicals within this subendothelial space where oxidation of the LDL is felt most likely to occur. Beta-carotene has also been shown to protect against LDL cholesterol oxidation; however, this effect seems to be negated in smokers.

With these findings in mind, researchers then went ahead to see if patients with higher antioxidant levels in their bodies truly had less cardiovascular disease. There have been several major epidemiological studies, as well as placebo-controlled clinical trials, that have demonstrated that an increased level of antioxidants does offer increased protection against coronary artery disease.[7]

EPIDEMIOLOGIC STUDIES

1. Two early studies in the United Kingdom reported that those individuals who had the greatest consumption of fruits and vegetables (foods that contain antioxidants) had a significantly decreased risk for vascular disease.[8,9]

2. Gey reported findings from 11 European countries where individuals with the highest vitamin E levels had the lowest incidence of cardiovascular mortality.[10]

3. Verlangieri reported a study in the United States that again showed those individuals who consumed greater amounts of fruits and vegetables had less cardiovascular mortality.[11]

CASE-CONTROL STUDIES

1. Riemersma showed that patients with angina had lower vitamin E levels than normal subjects.[12]

2. Ramirez and Flowers showed that those patients with coronary artery disease had the lowest levels of vitamin C when they were compared to normal subjects.[13]

PROSPECTIVE STUDIES

1. The Nurses Health Study, which followed over 87,000 nurses, showed that those individuals who had the highest level of vitamin E had the lowest incidence of coronary artery disease. There was also a 22 percent decreased risk of coronary artery disease and a 40 percent decreased risk of stroke in those individuals who had the highest levels of beta-carotene. The overall risk of cardiovascular disease significantly improved in the group that took supplements of vitamin E and beta-carotene for more than two years.[14,15,16]

2. In the Physicians Health Study, which followed 39,000 health care professionals, those who ingested 50 milligrams of beta-carotene had a 50 percent decreased incidence of major cardiovascular events. Also, those who had the highest levels of vitamin E showed the lowest risk of vascular disease. The improvement in overall risk of cardiovascular disease was seen more strongly in vitamin supplement users.[17]

3. The HANES-I study showed a significant reduction in cardiovascular events in those who took vitamin C supplementation.[18]

DOUBLE-BLIND, PLACEBO-CONTROLLED, CLINICAL TRIALS

1. The alpha-tocopherol (vitamin E), beta-carotene, cancer-prevention study observed 29,000 Finnish male smokers and found there was no effect on coronary artery disease by beta-carotene or vitamin E. This

demonstrates the fact that there is a definite negation of any beneficial effect of antioxidants in smokers.[19]

2. Howard Hodis studied 156 men who had previously undergone coronary artery bypass surgery. He followed them for more than two years and documented a decrease in coronary artery progression via angiography (injection of dye into the arteries) in those individuals who were taking vitamin E supplementation. In fact, a subgroup that was not only taking vitamin E supplements but also lowered LDL cholesterol to below 100 had an on-average clearing (actual improvement) of their coronary arteries.[20]

3. Dexter Morris reported in the Journal of the American Medical Association his study of 1,899 men with elevated lipids which showed a protective effect against developing coronary artery disease if they had high levels of serum carotenoids. Again, smokers did not experience the same beneficial effect as nonsmokers.[21]

4. In the Cambridge Heart Antioxidant Study, Nigel Stephens randomized 2,002 patients with angiographically proven coronary artery disease. Half received a placebo and the other half received either 400 or 800 International Units (IU) of vitamin E. These patients were then followed for an average of 18 months. The patients receiving the vitamin E supplement had 77 percent fewer nonfatal heart attacks than those taking the placebo. There was no significant difference between those patients taking 400 or 800 IU of vitamin E. These were astounding results since all of these patients had fairly advanced coronary artery disease. The authors concluded that the antioxidant effect of the vitamin E might actually stabilize these established plaques. The final event that leads to a heart attack is when one of these plaques ruptures away from the wall of the artery. A clot will then form at the site of rupture, and together with the plaque, it actually blocks the artery. The area of rupture always seems to occur in this layer of oxidized LDL. Antioxidants seem to play a protective role against coronary artery disease in two ways: They help prevent the initial formation of the plaque, and they also stabilize the plaque in advanced coronary artery disease.[22]

PRACTICAL CLINICAL APPLICATIONS

How do practicing clinicians apply the principles learned from these studies? Most research scientists are apparently going to guard their opinions until the evidence becomes overwhelming. This may be too late for many of us. I believe there is already overwhelming evidence in the medical literature that supports the use of nutritional supplements as a way to help prevent and reduce the risk of both heart attack and stroke.

In the August 7, 1997, issue of the New England Journal of Medicine, Marco Diaz, MD, wrote a review article called, "Antioxidants and Atherosclerotic Heart Disease." He concludes that antioxidants may very well reduce the risk of atherosclerosis by helping produce LDL resistance to oxidative modification and thus reduce the inflammation of the artery and the initial phase of atherosclerosis (the fatty streak). He goes on to state there may be other mechanisms by which antioxidants help reduce the risk of nonfatal heart attacks. This is probably by stabilizing the plaque where it is most likely to rupture, which is in the oxidized, LDL-laden, foam cell layer of the plaque. It may also reduce the size of the plaque. This means even individuals who have significantly advanced hardening of the arteries would benefit from supplementation with antioxidants.[23]

Medical researchers have a tendency to try to find a "magic bullet" with each disease process. Perhaps this is because we are so pharmaceutically oriented.

Medical researchers have a tendency to try to find a "magic bullet" with each disease process. Perhaps this is because we are so pharmaceutically oriented. However, this is inappropriate when it comes to nutritional supplements. Nutritional supplements are not drugs but nutrients that we should be getting from our food but at significantly higher levels than we can obtain from our food. One of the basic principles you need to remember is that all antioxidants and their supporting nutrients act synergistically. Given this fact, it is amazing how often there is a significant positive finding in these studies when only one nutrient is examined.

Vitamin C is water soluble and is the most important antioxidant in protecting LDL cholesterol within the plasma. Vitamin C also regenerates vitamin E. Vitamin E is lipid soluble and actually incorporates itself within the LDL cholesterol particle. Therefore, it is the best protector against the oxidation of

LDL cholesterol, even within the wall of the artery. Mixed carotenoids, alpha lipoic acid, and many other antioxidants also incorporate themselves within the LDL particle. Thus, they offer further protection against modification by excess free radicals.

Intracellular antioxidants, such as glutathione and its precursor N-acetyl L-cysteine, are very important within the cell. All these antioxidants are important in keeping the free radicals that are produced in balance. Additionally, in order for all of these antioxidants to function at an optimal level, there must be adequate levels of antioxidant minerals (selenium, copper, zinc, and manganese) and vitamin B cofactors (vitamins B1, B2, B6, B12, and folic acid). These nutrients are needed in the enzymatic reactions of the antioxidants. If these nutrients are not available in sufficient amounts, antioxidants are cannot function at their optimal level. Therefore, when you finally become convinced you must take nutritional supplements to protect your health, you must realize that the biochemical atmosphere must be complete and balanced for each cell to perform at its optimal level. Synergy (teamwork) is a major key when taking nutritional supplements.

I believe that cardiologists as a group are the most informed when it comes to the potential health benefits of antioxidant supplementation. The evidence in medical literature is just too strong to continue to ignore. If you have adequate levels of antioxidants, the bad cholesterol (LDL) is no longer bad. I still encourage all my patients to keep their cholesterol as low as possible, and especially LDL cholesterol. I am very committed to keeping LDL cholesterol in my patients with coronary artery disease below 100. The medical literature has established the fact that this decreases the risk of further heart attacks. However, it is my belief that the reason for this benefit is the fact that there is just less LDL cholesterol available to become oxidized. The most important recommendation is to make sure that my cardiac patients are taking adequate antioxidants. I feel that by doing both (lowering LDL cholesterol and adding antioxidants), my patients will have the greatest benefit.

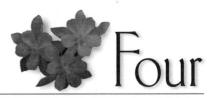Four

Homocysteine
THE NEW KID ON THE BLOCK

Kilmer McCully, MD, described a theory of atherosclerosis in 1969. Dr. McCully, a young pathology instructor at Harvard Medical School, became intrigued by two different cases involving children who had a rare genetic defect called homocystinuria. Children with this disease have a very high level of homocysteine in their blood because they lack the proper enzymes to break it down into a harmless substance. They had hardening of the arteries much like an 80-year-old with severe atherosclerosis. Both of these boys died of heart attacks. That is significant since one of these boys was eight years old and the other was ten. Most children with homocystinuria do not even reach their teenage years but instead die of coronary artery disease or stroke. This led Dr. McCully to theorize that maybe mildly elevated homocysteine levels over a longer period of time could be involved in the process of atherosclerosis in everyone.

His theory was initially met with some degree of enthusiasm. By the mid-1970s, however, his research funds began to dry up, and studies on cholesterol began to take center stage. In 1979, he actually lost his appointment at Harvard and spent the next two years looking for a job. His homocysteine theory was actively criticized and almost forgotten.[1]

Meir Stampfer, a professor of epidemiology and nutrition at the Harvard School of Public Health, revived the interest in homocysteine. He looked at the blood levels of homocysteine in 15,000 physicians who were involved in the Physicians' Health Study.[2] Stampfer reported that even mildly elevated levels of homocysteine were directly related to an increased risk of heart disease. Those men who had the highest level of homocysteine had three times the risk of developing a heart attack when compared with those who had the lower levels. This was the first large study that showed the possibility that homocysteine might be an independent risk factor for heart disease. This was a major turning point in the research of homocysteine, and the interest in McCully's original theory was revitalized.

Since the mid-1980s, there have been well over 40 major clinical studies that have all demonstrated that homocysteine, even at levels once considered normal, is associated with a definite increased risk of both heart attack and stroke.

WHAT IS HOMOCYSTEINE?

Homocysteine is a sulfur-containing amino acid involved in the metabolism of methionine, an essential amino acid. Methionine is most commonly found in meats, eggs, and dairy products. During normal metabolism within the body, it is broken down into homocysteine, which in turn is broken down into cysteine (which is harmless) or sometimes actually turned back into methionine again. The enzymes needed to turn homocysteine back into methionine require vitamin B12 as a cofactor and folic acid as a substrate. Homocysteine may also be broken down into cysteine, but this enzymatic reaction requires vitamin B6. Don't let this confuse you. Just remember: You must have adequate levels of folic acid, vitamin B6, and vitamin B12 for homocysteine levels to remain in a safe range.

When homocysteine levels increase, there is a direct toxic or irritative effect to the endothelium. This is probably one of the most important causes of inflammation of the endothelium. This leads to either an actual disruption or dysfunction of the endothelium. One of the proposed mechanisms of this damage has been related to oxidative stress. Once the lining of our arteries is damaged, there seems to be an attraction of LDL cholesterol, which may act as a bandage, trying to help heal the endothelium.[3] This repair mechanism may actually prove to be more harmful than good. Remember the role of the oxidized LDL in atherosclerosis from the previous chapter.

CLINICAL STUDIES

From the Framingham cohort study, Jacob Selhub, MD, reported in the New England Journal of Medicine that there was a significantly increased risk of carotid artery stenosis (narrowing of the two large arteries supplying blood to the brain) in those individuals who had higher levels of homocysteine.[4] There seemed to be a continuous rise in the risk of carotid stenosis as the level of homocysteine increased. In other words, there was no specific threshold at which the problem started. The higher the level of homocysteine,

These authors estimated that 10 to 15 percent of every heart attack and stroke in this country were caused just by elevated homocysteine levels. This means that somewhere between 150,000 and 225,000 hearts attacks a year are related solely to elevated homocysteine levels.

the worse the risk; or, in other words, the lower the level, the better. Dr. Selhub made another interesting observation: Most all of the patients who had high levels of homocysteine had deficiencies in vitamin B6, vitamin B12, and folic acid. Furthermore, when these three nutrients were given in supplementation, the majority of the patients' homocysteine levels returned to a safer level rather quickly.

Another large prospective study out of Tromso, Norway, showed that the higher the homocysteine level, the greater the risk of developing a heart attack.[5] What were once considered normal levels for homocysteine were now being shown to be dangerous. Homocysteine seemed to be as strong a risk, if not actually greater, of vascular disease as cholesterol, hypertension, and smoking. Of even more concern was the fact that when elevated levels of homocysteine were found in patients who also had one or more of these other major risk factors (hypertension, elevated cholesterol, or smoking), the risk of vascular disease increased dramatically. It has become very evident that the lower our homocysteine level, the better.

In the Journal of the American Medical Association, Boushey and associates reviewed 27 previously published studies relating homocysteine to various forms of vascular disease. These authors concluded that increased levels of homocysteine were an independent risk factor for coronary artery disease, stroke, and peripheral vascular disease. They also reported that the overwhelming majority of these patients who had elevated levels of homocysteine also had nutritional deficiencies of folic acid, vitamin B6, and vitamin B12. These authors estimated that 10 to 15 percent of every heart attack and stroke in this country were caused just by elevated homocysteine levels.[6] This means that somewhere between 150,000 and 225,000 hearts attacks a year are related solely to elevated homocysteine levels. More than nine million people with vascular disease in this country can blame homocysteine as the culprit for their disease. After researching this subject, I believe these estimates are even on the conservative side.

The medical literature also points out that there is a group of individuals – probably 10 to 12 percent of the population – who have minor genetic defects (not full-blown homocystinuria) that make it more difficult for them to break down homocysteine.[7] These people are obviously at an even higher risk of developing vascular disease. The interesting finding was that when these individuals were given higher levels of folic acid (1,000 micrograms [mcg] daily), even their homocysteine levels came down into a safer range. Some studies found that if you give the general population 1,000 mcg of folic acid along with vitamins B6 and B12 in supplementation, 92 percent of the homocysteine levels would fall into the safer range.[8] The medical literature is also showing us that the lower your homocysteine level, the better. Everyone who takes vitamin B6, vitamin B12, and folic acid in supplementation at these recommended levels will significantly lower their homocysteine level. Even individuals who have homocysteine levels that are considered normal will benefit by taking these nutrients. Remember: you want your homocysteine level as low as possible.

Data from the Framingham Study and throughout all the other studies show that the individuals with the lowest levels of folic acid, vitamin B6, and vitamin B12 had the highest levels of homocysteine. The researchers concluded that elevated homocysteine levels were the first sign of folic acid deficiency. So why don't we recommend that everyone in this country just take folic acid, vitamin B6, and vitamin B12 in supplementation? Could the natural bias that physicians and the medical community in general has against nutritional supplements be affecting our decisions in this area. The government instead has required the manufacturers of our cereals to add folic acid to our cereals rather than recommending folic acid supplements. But isn't this actually a means of supplementation? Why doesn't the government just recommend supplementation with folic acid, B6, and B12?

There have been two major studies in the past couple of years that will shed some light on this approach. Geraldine Cuskelly reported the effect of dietary folic acid on red-cell folate level (much better than the serum level of folate) in the March 1996 issue of British Lancet. Pregnant women who have good levels of folic acid have been shown to decrease the risk of neural tube defects (spina bifida, hydrocephalus, etc.) in their babies by as much as 70 percent. The United Kingdom has advised physicians to recommend to women in their child-bearing years to either eat foods high in folic acid, fortified with folic acid, or to take at least 400 mcg of folic acid in supplementation. It was demonstrated, however, that eating foods high in folic acid was relatively ineffective in increasing folate status. Only those who took folic acid in supplementation or ate foods fortified with folic acid achieved the desired level of folic acid, which gave optimal protection to their child. They concluded by advising women that consuming folate-rich foods may not offer optimal protection against neural tube defects in their children.[9]

Judith Brown reported a similar study in the February 19, 1997, issue of the Journal of the American Medical Association in which red-cell folate levels were measured. Red-cell folate levels of less than 340 nmol/L (this is the means by which folic acid in a red blood cell is measured) showed an eight-fold increase in the risk of neural tube defects when compared with red-cell folate levels above 906 nmol/L. (It is interesting that this is the same level that offers the best protection against the buildup of homocysteine.)

Patients were divided into three groups: 1) *those who consumed foods high in folic acid*, 2) *those who consumed cereals fortified with folic acid*, and 3) *those who took folic acid supplements of 450 mcg daily*. Those individuals who achieved a red cell folate level of greater that 906 nmol/L were nearly exclusively found among the supplement users. Interestingly, they found those who also took vitamin C along with their folic acid had the highest levels of folate. They also concluded that a diet high in folic acid, even if it included cereals and grains fortified with folic acid, would not provide optimal protection against neural tube defects.[10]

In the lead article of the April 9, 1998, issue of the New England Journal of Medicine, Manuel R. Malinow, MD, et al. reported on the effect folic acid fortification had on homocysteine levels. It has been estimated that the level of folic acid fortification recommended by the Food and Drug Administration (140 micrograms of folic acid per 100 grams of cereal) would increase the level of

However, the pharmaceutical companies won't be taking out a full-page ad in USA Today to tell you about folic acid, vitamin B6, and vitamin B12. There is no money in it. Could that have been one of the main reasons Dr. McCully's research grants disappeared? There is definitely a lot more money in cholesterol-lowering drugs– billions more.

folic acid intake to somewhere between 80 and 120 micrograms per day. He concluded that the level of fortification of cereals with folic acid that had been recommended by the FDA did not have a significant effect on the plasma levels of homocysteine. This, in turn, was felt to not have any significant effect on vascular disease in this country. He believed that the level of supplementation for folic acid should be four to five times higher than those recommended by the FDA.[11]

These studies shed some light on the risk of elevated homocysteine. Increasing foods rich in folic acid and eating cereals fortified with folic acid is not enough. It is obvious to me that we need to be taking folic acid, vitamin B6, and vitamin B12 in supplementation to be assured of significantly decreasing this risk. Simply by taking 1,000 mcg of folic acid, 50 to 75 mcg of vitamin B12, and 25 mg of vitamin B6, we can potentially eliminate this risk factor altogether. Doesn't it seem logical to spend a few pennies a day to reduce the risk of the number one killer in America today by at least 15 percent? There really is no downside to this recommendation.

So why aren't physicians shouting this from the rooftops? Aren't they concerned about their patients' health? I don't believe that is the problem. Are they uninformed? Possibly. The medical literature is overwhelming in support of the use of supplementation as a way to decrease the inherent health risk of homocysteine. Cardiologists as a group appreciate the value of folic acid, vitamin B6, and vitamin B12 supplementation more than anyone else. However, the pharmaceutical companies won't be taking out a full-page ad in USA Today to tell you about folic acid, vitamin B6, and vitamin B12. There is no money in it. Could that have been one of the main reasons Dr. McCully's research grants disappeared? There is definitely a lot more money in cholesterol-lowering drugs – billions more.

The more I learn about the value of nutritional supplementation, the more I am learning about the economics of medicine. None of the physicians or their patients are uninformed about the value of lowering their cholesterol level. Why have so few people learned about the value of lowering their homocysteine level?

Had you even heard about homocysteine before reading this book? The difference between these two risk factors for cardiovascular disease – cholesterol and homocysteine – is money. Look at the ads you see on TV, in the newspaper, and in the magazines. Who is educating you on cholesterol? It is the same people who are educating the physicians. The pharmaceutical companies are the main educators of the health benefits of lowering cholesterol for both the physician and the public. Who benefits the most from an entire society becoming totally consumed about cholesterol? You guessed it, the pharmaceutical industry. Literally billions of dollars are spent each year on testing and treating for cholesterol. Who finances most of the studies on cholesterol-lowering drugs? I can honestly tell you there is rarely a week that goes by that at least one pharmaceutical representative doesn't come into my office to show me the results of the study their company has done on demonstrating the value of their cholesterol-lowering drug on heart disease. I have yet to have anyone come into my office to show me the benefits of testing and treating elevated homocysteine levels.

Such is the state of medicine today. Unless physicians are willing to become their patients' advocate, examine their own medical literature, and decide what is best for the health of their patients, things will not change.

Dr. Ross just wrote an article in the January 14, 1999, issue of the New England Journal of Medicine about the cause of atherosclerosis.[12] He states that atherosclerosis is an inflammatory disease of the arteries. That is right. It is not a disease of elevated cholesterol. He states that free radicals, oxidized LDL cholesterol, homocysteine, and even possibly some infectious agents cause an inflammation of the endothelium. This, in turn, causes either a disruption of the endothelium or a dysfunction of the endothelium. Then along comes the oxidized LDL cholesterol to try and patch up this damage somewhat like a Band-Aid. This apparent healing process actually sets up the progression of atherosclerosis. The amazing reality of this basic cause of the number one killer in the industrialized world – inflammation – is the fact that all of the root causes of the inflammation would be significantly reduced by the use of nutritional supplementation. Antioxidants lower the amount of oxidized LDL and the amount of free radicals. Folic acid, vitamin B6, and vitamin B12 significantly lower the risk of elevated homocysteine levels. As you will learn later in this book, nutritional supplements greatly improve our immune system. This would definitely decrease our risk of infection. However, you will only hear about these truths in books like this and maybe occasionally on shows like 20/20.

Nowhere is the economics of medicine more evident than when it comes to the treatment of congestive heart failure and cardiomyopathy. You will understand why I say this after you have read the next chapter.

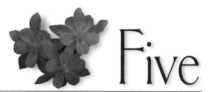 Five

Cardiomyopathy - New Hope

The heart is not a very complicated organ. It is essentially a muscle that pumps blood throughout the body. It also has its own electrical system, that allows it to beat in an efficient manner. There are valves that keep the blood flowing in the right direction. Coronary arteries provide the heart with an adequate amount of oxygen and nutrients to perform its job.

In the previous two chapters we have discussed hardening of the arteries. We will now focus on congestive heart failure and cardiomyopathy, which are diseases that involve the heart muscle itself. When the heart muscle becomes weak, it is not able to pump all the blood it receives from the body (through the venous system). Therefore, the blood backs up into the lungs. The lungs fill up with fluid and the patient essentially begins to drown. We call this congestive heart failure. Cardiomyopathy is simply a more severe form of congestive heart failure in that the heart is extremely weak and dilated.

There are several causes of congestive heart failure and cardiomyopathy. Hypertension, coronary artery disease, and viral infections of the heart are examples of just some of the causes. The standard medical treatment for this disease is diuretics, digitalis, angiotensin-converting enzyme inhibitors (known more commonly as ACE inhibitors), and more recently beta-blockers. Patients with cardiomyopathy usually have only minimal improvement through these traditional medical regimens. The only option for many of these patients is a heart transplant.

Heart muscle cells have a high-energy requirement. Biochemical research in recent years has demonstrated that the heart muscle in patients with congestive heart failure and cardiomyopathy is deficient in a largely unknown nutrient called Coenzyme Q10 (CoQ10). The more severe the heart failure, the more severe the depletion of CoQ10. This has been a consistent finding no matter what the underlying cause of the heart failure. There is some speculation among researchers that CoQ10 deficiency may well be an underlying cause of heart failure; others consider it a secondary phenomenon.[1]

WHAT IS COENZYME Q10?

CoQ10, or ubiquinone, is a fat-soluble vitamin or vitamin-like substance that also has antioxidant activity. CoQ10 is found in small amounts in a variety of foods (organ meats, beef, soy oil, sardines, mackerel, and peanuts). The body also has the ability to make CoQ10 from the amino acid tyrosine. However, this is a 17-step process that requires at least eight vitamins and several trace minerals. A deficiency in any one of these nutrients can hinder the body's production of CoQ10.

Coenzymes as a group are cofactors essential for a large number of enzymatic reactions within the body. CoQ10 is the cofactor for at least three very important enzymes used within the mitochondria of the cell. The mitochondria is essentially the battery of the cell. This is where cell energy is produced. Mitochondrial enzymes are essential for the production of the high-energy phosphate called adenosine triphosphate (ATP), upon which all cellular function depends. Remember: The mitochondria is where the oxidative process occurs. Not only is this where energy is created, but the by-products are free radicals.

CoQ10 was first isolated from the beef heart mitochondria by Frederick Crane, MD, in 1957. In 1958, Karl Folkers, MD, and coworkers at Merck, Inc., determined the exact chemical structure of CoQ10 and began synthesizing it. In the mid-1970s, the Japanese perfected the technology and are now able to produce large amounts of pure CoQ10.

COQ10 DEFICIENCY AND HEART FAILURE

The normal blood levels of CoQ10 have been well established by numerous investigators. Significantly decreased amounts of CoQ10 have been noted in several diseases. The deficient levels of CoQ10 have been established most clearly, however, in congestive heart failure and cardiomyopathy. There seems to be a direct correlation between the severity of heart failure and the severity of the depletion of CoQ10. CoQ10 deficiency can be caused by 1) *poor dietary intake*, 2) *impairment of the body's ability to synthesize CoQ10*, and 3) *excessive utilization of CoQ10 by the body or a combination of these factors*. I believe that in cardiomyopathy the main cause of the depletion of CoQ10 is because the heart-muscle cell is over utilizing it just trying to compensate for its weakened state. It simply is using up its fuel source.

Coenzyme Q10 has been noted by several investigators to be significantly depleted in the blood and heart muscle of patients with heart failure. Investigators in the early 1980s began supplementing these patients with CoQ10 to see if there would be any improvement in their clinical situation. These clinical trials were made possible by the availability of pure CoQ10 in large quantities from pharmaceutical companies in Japan and the ability to directly measure the level of CoQ10 within the blood and tissue.

Several clinical trials have now been done comparing the effect of adding CoQ10 in supplementation to the patients' medication with cardiomyopathy or congestive heart failure and comparing them with those who took a placebo. There have been no fewer than nine placebo-controlled clinical trials in the world that have evaluated the treatment of heart failure with CoQ10. There have been eight international symposia on the biomedical and clinical aspects of CoQ10. During these symposia, more than 300 papers were presented from more than 200 physicians and scientists from 18 different countries. The largest of these studies was the Italian multicenter trial by Baggio and associates involving 2,664 patients with heart failure.[2] In the United States the leading investigator has been Dr. Peter Langsjoen, who is not only a cardiologist but also a biochemist. He has reported several studies in the medical literature in regards to the use of CoQ10 in cardiomyopathy.

All of these studies have confirmed the effectiveness of CoQ10 in congestive heart failure and cardiomyopathy, along with its safety. The patients continued their conventional medical treatment and CoQ10 was added to their regimen. Comparison was made with those who either received placebo or conventional medical therapy. Heart function was determined by the percentage of blood the heart was able to pump during a contraction (ejection fraction). In most cases this was established by echocardiography, which is a sound-wave study of the heart. Clinical improvement was determined by using the New York Heart Association (NYHA) classification for functional capacity.

The function of the heart showed gradual and sustained improvement in muscle contraction as noted by improved ejection fraction, heart-wall motion, and heart size. The overwhelming majority of patients had improvement in their symptoms of fatigue, chest pain, shortness of breath, exercise ability, and palpitations. The improvement in some patients was dramatic, with both heart size and function returning to normal. The patients who started CoQ10 shortly after developing their disease seemed to have the most dramatic improvement. The patients who had their heart disease for a longer time improved but usually not to the same degree. The individuals with the worst heart failure actually had the greatest percentage of improvement. These amazing results were coupled with the fact that CoQ10 did not create any serious side effects, even at the highest doses. An eight-year, follow-up study has shown that these patients have maintained these improvements. In other words, the use of CoQ10 was found not only to be safe but effective.

TABLE I
CLINICAL TRIALS WITH COENZYME Q10 AND CARDIOMYOPATHY

REFERENCE	SUBJECTS	RESULTS
Langsjoen, 1988 3	88 patients with cardiomyopathy	Statistically significant improvement was seen in 75% to 85% in two cardiac parameters.
Langsjoen, 1990 4	137 patients with cardiomyopathy	The survival rates for all 137 patients treated with CoQ10 was 75% at 46 months. This is very significant when compared with 25% at 36 months in patients on conventional therapy without COQ10.

REFERENCE	SUBJECTS	RESULTS
Langsjoen, 1990 5	143 patients with cardiomyopathy	Given 100 mg CoQ10 mean ejection fraction of 44% rose to 60% in six months and stabilized at that level, with 84% of the patients showing this improvement; this was sustained over the six years of this trial.
Manzoli, 1990 6	30 patients with cardiomyopathy	In 47% of the patients, symptoms improved within two months with 100 mg of CoQ10.
Davini, 1992 7	63 patients with cardiomyopathy	Double-blind placebo trial. Those patients who received CoQ10 had a significant improvement in functional capacity and in the strength of their heart.
Mortensen, 1993 8	45 patients with cardiomyopathy	Two-thirds of the patients had significant improvement while taking 100 mg CoQ10.
Langsjoen, 1994 9	424 patients with cardiovascular disease	According to the American Heart Association functional scale, on 75 to 600 mg CoQ10, 58% improved by one class; 28% improved by two classes.

Soja and Mortensen (1997) reported in the medical literature a meta-analysis of seven studies they reviewed to investigate the effect of CoQ10 in patients with congestive heart failure. These studies showed a consistent improvement of heart function in almost all parameters in those patients taking CoQ10.

CLINICAL APPLICATIONS

There are more than 20,000 patients under the age of 65 who are eligible for a heart transplant. There are many more over 65 who have cardiomyopathy but are ineligible to be on the heart transplant list. They receive maximal medical treatment, but most are still totally disabled. Only about 1 out of 10 who are eligible for a heart transplant will actually receive one. The other nine will most likely end up dying from their disease. The cost of a heart transplant is approximately $250,000. There are hundreds of thousands of individuals who have congestive heart failure who are not able to function normally because of their disease but who are not bad enough to be on a heart transplant list.

I believe that all individuals with cardiomyopathy and congestive heart failure should be placed on good doses of pharmaceutical-grade CoQ10 (100 to 400 mg per day). This should be given in addition to their traditional medical treatments, not as a replacement.

Doctors Folkers and Langsjoen reported a study in the medical literature in 1992 which I believe brings all of this to an obvious conclusion.[10] They placed 11 exemplary transplant candidates on CoQ10, all of whom improved. Three of these patients improved from NYHA class IV to class I. That is going from the worst classification to the best classification under the New York Heart Association guide. Four improved from class III-IV to class II. Two others improved from class III to class I. These authors concluded that with these case histories and the substantial clinical trials already reported in the medical literature showing proof of efficacy and safety, patients with end-stage heart failure awaiting transplantation should receive CoQ10. With the improvement these 11 patients had, they all would have been taken off the heart transplant list.

This is a prime example of a natural vitamin and antioxidant shown in several clinical trials to be effective and safe. It is bionutrition at its best. When the heart muscle is weakened – for whatever reason – it places an increased demand on the nutrients the heart cell needs to create energy. Because of excessive utilization of these nutrients, the heart muscle eventually becomes depleted. The most important of these nutrients is CoQ10. When this nutrient is given in supplementation, the weakened heart muscle is simply able to replenish its stores of CoQ10. This allows the heart muscle to generate more energy and compensate for its weakened state. It is important to note again that CoQ10 is used in support of the traditional medical treatment and not in place of it. This is not alternative medicine. It is medicine at its best because we are supporting the host (our bodies). Many patients improved so much that they were able to come off several of their medications during these clinical trials. However, the patient is not cured of his or her underlying heart disease. The clinical studies show that when supplementation of CoQ10 is discontinued, the heart function slowly reverts back to its previously poor level.

WHY DON'T PHYSICIANS RECOMMEND COQ10?

Here we have a life-threatening disease in which there is very little hope for improvement with traditional medical therapy. The cost of taking CoQ10 in supplementation is about a dollar a day, less than the $250,000 heart transplant for which most of these patients are waiting. There have never been shown any side effects or problems in trying to use CoQ10 in supplementation. Most of the studies show there is improvement within four months. So, then, why don't physicians recommend a trial of CoQ10 to their cardiomyopathy patients?

I have never heard a discussion of the use of CoQ10 at any medical meeting or with any cardiologist. I have never had any cardiologist place any of my patients with congestive heart failure or cardiomyopathy on CoQ10. In fact, a recent survey showed that only 1% of the cardiologists in the United States recommends CoQ10 to their patients with cardiomyopathy. After reviewing these studies, I am simply amazed at the unwillingness of the medical profession to offer supplementation of CoQ10 to their patients. It is not as if we have any good alternative therapy. I don't consider a heart transplant a great option, even if you are able to get one.

Some physicians hesitate to recommend CoQ10 to their patients because it has not been approved by the FDA. Physicians must remember CoQ10 is a natural product. Therefore, it cannot be patented. (A special-use patent can be obtained, but, as long as the product can be purchased over the counter, it has no value.) Pharmaceutical companies are not going to spend the millions of dollars needed to get a drug or natural product approved by the FDA if there is no economic incentive. It is very costly for a company to promote the use of its medication by physicians. Physicians are pharmaceutically trained. We know drugs; we don't

BIONUTRITION

know much about natural products. As much as we hate to admit it, the pharmaceutical sales representatives who come to our offices daily control much of what we learn in regards to new treatments. I have not seen a pharmaceutical sales representative show me one of these studies on CoQ10 supplementation in patients with cardiomyopathy. We need to evaluate the medical literature on our own when it comes to the use of CoQ10. Then we need to begin utilizing it in our own practice. I have been involved with no less than twelve patients who have been taken off the heart transplant list since they started taking CoQ10 in supplementation.

Physicians must become their patients' advocates. We need to learn and understand how natural products can help our patients. There is a basic principle here that cannot be emphasized too much. When we support the natural functioning of the body and try to elevate this function to its optimal level, then and only then have we done everything possible for the patient.

A REAL-LIFE STORY

A high school friend who grew up with me in a small South Dakota town came to my office over a year ago. He was complaining of shortness of breath, fatigue, and heart palpitations. He had always been very athletic and very active. He told me these symptoms had come on over a two-to-three-month period of time.

After a thorough evaluation in the hospital, we found that he had developed a serious cardiomyopathy. He related to me in retrospect that he had developed a serious, flu-like illness during the early spring. He most likely had viral myocarditis that damaged the heart extensively. His ejection fraction upon admission to the hospital was only 17 percent (normal is usually 50 to 70 percent). The ejection fraction is a measurement of how strongly the heart contracts. The cardiologist placed him on traditional medical therapy, and his ejection fraction improved to 23 percent. Anytime the ejection fraction is below 30 percent, the patient should consider being placed on a heart transplant list. He was able to return home but unable to return to work. His heartbeat was very irregular and his heart was filled with blood clots. He was placed on blood thinners, and eventually we were able to convert the rhythm of his heart back to a normal sinus rhythm.

It was at this time that I became familiar with the studies on CoQ10 supplementation in patients with cardiomyopathy. I started him on a complete and balanced nutritional supplement and added 200 mg of pharmaceutical-grade CoQ10. His ejection fraction at this time was still around 25 percent. After four months on this program, he was riding his bike again and feeling significantly better. I told him I thought we should reevaluate his heart. He agreed and we found that his ejection fraction had improved to 51 percent, within the normal range. I shared this information with his cardiologist. Needless to say, he was definitely surprised. He wanted to recheck my patient and do another echocardiogram in his office. To his amazement, my patient's ejection fraction was 58 percent. My patient was quite excited. He has returned to full-time work and is back doing his workout program. He still has his heart disease, but he is not on any heart transplant list.

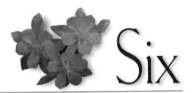

Six

Chemoprevention and Cancer

There will be more than 1,359,000 new cases of cancer diagnosed in the United States this year. Approximately 550,000 patients will die from cancer this year. In spite of nearly $25 billion spent on cancer research in the past 20 years, cancer deaths have actually increased over that same time period. This has raised a major concern among researchers and clinicians alike. There is a call to rethink our approach to cancer prevention and treatment. If there has been any improvement in cancer risk, it seems to be with the ability to detect some cancers sooner, such as mammography for the detection of breast cancer and PSA tests for prostate cancer. In this chapter, we will discuss some of the most recent advances in cancer research and show you how these may help you personally lower your risk of developing cancer.

It seems that everything we do or eat these days causes cancer. Excessive exposure to sunlight increases the risk of skin cancer. Asbestos workers have increased risk of developing an unusual form of lung cancer called mesothelioma. Smoking and secondary smoke are the main reasons lung cancer is the leading cause of death due to cancer (more than 158,000 deaths in 1996 alone). Radiation, charcoal-broiled steaks, too much fat in our diet, saccharin, along with numerous chemicals can also increase our risk of cancer. These are referred to in medical literature and the media as carcinogens, or those things that increase our risk of developing cancer.

Since the first report that chimney sweeps have an increased risk of scrotal cancer because of their exposure to soot, we have become more and more afraid of our environment. Our bodies are being exposed to far more chemicals than any previous generation. The Environmental Protection Agency has estimated there are well over 60,000 chemicals in commercial use today, and they are increasing at the rate of a thousand per year. What is the one common denominator all of these carcinogens have in common? You guessed it – they all increase oxidative stress. This is the key to understanding possible new strategies for fighting cancer.

OXIDATIVE STRESS AS THE CAUSE OF CANCER

There has been growing medical evidence that when excess free radicals are allowed to exist near the nucleus of a cell, there is significant damage to the DNA of the cell.[1] If this damage is not rapidly repaired, this free-radical damage may lead to actual mutation of the cell's DNA. This mutation is then passed on as the cell replicates. When there is further oxidative stress to the DNA of the cell, the DNA is damaged further. The cell will then begin to grow out of control and take on a life of its own. It develops the ability to spread from one part of the body to another (metastasis). Thus, it becomes a true cancer.[2]

Most researchers now agree that the development of cancer is not an event but rather a multistage process that takes decades to unfold. More and more researchers are beginning to realize that it is repeated damage to the DNA by these excess free radicals over 10, 20, even 30 years that eventually leads to cancer.

Donald Malins, MD, a biochemist from Seattle, has reported a new method for identifying structural changes in the DNA of breast tissue. By using an instrument that bounces infrared radiation off the DNA and analyzing the signals via a sophisticated computer, he has been able to follow the structural changes to the DNA caused by these free radicals. He was able to note significant changes within the structure of the DNA as he followed normal breast tissue all the way to actual metastatic breast cancer and all the stages in-between. As mentioned previously, this process of going from normal breast tissue to full-blown metastatic breast cancer takes decades. Dr. Malins believes oxidative stress caused this predictable damage to the DNA and eventually led to the formation of breast cancer. He also believes that cancer is not so much the result of dysfunctional genes as it is the result of genetic damage caused by these highly reactive free radicals. He feels that some individuals may be more genetically predisposed to this free radical damage, which would account for familial tendencies of certain cancer risks. However, it is the free-radical damage that is the cause of cancer and not the genetic abnormality.[3]

Kelvin Davies, a biochemist from the Department of Biochemistry at Albany Medical College, wrote an extensive review article on oxidative stress.[1] He explained how extensive damage can occur to the DNA of a cell via excess free radicals. He was even able to identify which chains of the DNA are damaged most frequently. This damage actually causes mutation of the genetic code within the DNA. For the past 25 years, researchers have been focused on the fact that abnormal genes are the driving force behind all cancers. Here again, Kelvin Davies and other researchers are starting to believe that maybe some genes are just more vulnerable to oxidative stress than others. This again would explain the familial pattern of many types of cancer.

Physicians usually diagnose cancer in its last stages. By the time cancer is advanced enough to cause symptoms or to show up on an x-ray, it has been developing for more than 20 to 30 years. Doctors get out their big guns of aggressive surgery, chemotherapy, and radiation, only to realize that often there is not much that can be done to help these patients.

The last time I diagnosed lung cancer in one of my patients, the oncologist consulted the patient and recommended chemotherapy. He said that he could get his cancer into remission about 40 percent of the time if he took the chemotherapy he recommended. My patient was somewhat encouraged by those statistics until he asked the oncologist just exactly what he meant by remission. The oncologist informed my patient that if he could get his cancer into remission, he could extend his life by about three months. Needless to say, this was not exactly what my patient wanted to hear.

My mother was diagnosed with a high-grade brain tumor, and I remember very clearly when the radiation therapist consulted. He stated that he had a one-percent chance of extending her life if she took the radiation treatments. My mother went through those treatments against my wishes. She died six months later. Unfortunately, this is all too familiar a story with many of our cancer patients. We may extend their life a few months or even a year or so. However, the suffering we put our patients through for those marginal benefits seems cruel.

At present, we are losing the battle against cancer. As I illustrated above, by the time we diagnose cancer it is usually too late for the patient. We need to be attacking cancer at a much earlier stage in its development if we are going to have any chance of decreasing the number of deaths caused by cancer. Understanding the role of oxidative stress in the development of cancer offers us a host of new possibilities in cancer prevention and treatment.

DO ANTIOXIDANTS DECREASE THE RISK OF CANCER?

It would seem logical that if oxidative stress were the cause of cancer, then antioxidants used to bring these free radicals back into balance would lower the risk of cancer. Cancer researcher Dr. Gladys Block reviewed 172 epidemiological studies from around the world that had been done looking at an individual's diet and how it related to cancer. There was an almost universal and consistent finding: Those individuals who had the highest intake of fruits and vegetables (our main source of antioxidants) showed a huge protective effect against almost every kind of cancer. Those who ate the most fruits and vegetables, as compared to those who ate the least, had a two-to three-fold risk decrease in almost every type of cancer. Dr. Bruce Ames, a leading cancer researcher, stated in an interview in the Journal of the American Medical Association that those individuals who consume the least amount of fruits and vegetables have twice the cancer risk of those who consume the most fruits and vegetables.[4]

By merely consuming the recommended five-to-seven servings of fruits and vegetables on a daily basis, we are able to significantly decrease our risk of almost every type of cancer. Fruits and vegetables are the primary source of antioxidants. One of the principles you will hear me promote over and over is the fact that if you choose to use nutritional supplements, you should be supplementing a good diet, not a bad diet. The start toward decreasing your risk of cancer is to eat a high-fiber, low-fat diet largely made up of fruits and vegetables.

CHEMOPREVENTION OF CANCER

As we begin to understand the root cause of cancer, many different therapeutic options become available. Since cancer is a multistage process that takes decades to develop from the first mutation of the DNA by free radicals to the point that the tumor is actually malignant, there are several opportunities to intervene in this process. In the earliest stages, we see the changes are primarily within the DNA nucleus itself. The mutations that occur via the free-radical attack on the DNA are passed on to each subsequent cell as it replicates. Eventually, because of further free-radical damage to the cell, a precancerous tumor develops. This is the first practical level that can be evaluated clinically. The final stage is the development of a malignancy or cancer which has the ability to spread from one part of the body to another.

Chemoprevention is focused on preventing the cancer from developing in its earliest stages. If we have enough antioxidants available, oxidative stress will not occur in the first place. The DNA is essentially protected from the initial damage. If this is not possible, chemoprevention is aimed at reversing the damage that has already occurred to the cell. The body has the amazing ability to heal itself if it has the proper level of micronutrients available. This is the very basis of bionutrition.

CHEMOPREVENTION: PHASE I

The first strategy in the prevention of cancer is the elimination of exposure to carcinogens.

1. Cigarette smoke is the most potent carcinogen to which many of us are exposed. The tobacco industry is finally starting to admit to the general public what physicians have known for a long time. Nicotine is one of the most addictive drugs with which we must deal. I have a much more difficult time getting patients to quit smoking than I do to quit drinking. There is a tremendous increase in the amount of free radicals in the bodies of smokers. Even though it is to a lesser extent, secondary smoke is also an important factor in oxidative stress. (5)

2. Excessive exposure to sunlight is a well-known carcinogen. Studies are now demonstrating beyond any shadow of doubt that oxidative stress caused by sunlight is what actually leads to skin cancer. Have you ever wondered why we are seeing such an increase in skin cancer, despite the fact that most of us are using sunscreens? It is not because of the increasing ozone hole. You see, our sunscreens are primarily protecting us from UVB sunlight, which is responsible for causing us to sunburn. However, we are not being protected from the UVA sunlight responsible for causing oxidative stress in our skin, which leads to skin cancer. So what we have been doing is putting on our sunscreen to protect us from sunburn, and then spending more time out in the sun than we normally

would. This allows us to expose our skin to significantly more UVA sunlight and increase the risk of cancer. You need to be using a sunscreen that protects against both UVA and UVB ultraviolet light. It is important to remember that sunlight is a great source of vitamin D. We just don't need to overdue it.

3. Excessive fat intake with a meal is known to induce oxidative stress, especially when there are inadequate amounts of antioxidants within that meal. These may be provided in some degree by fruits and vegetables, but clinical studies demonstrate that antioxidant supplements taken with a fatty meal actually prevent this source of oxidative stress.

4. Other carcinogens that need to be avoided include radiation, pesticides, herbicides, asbestos, charcoal, soot, and so forth.[6]

CHEMOPREVENTION: PHASE II

It is not possible to avoid being exposed to all of these carcinogens and chemicals that are in the environment. We must still live in this world. Living in a bubble would not be very attractive or much fun. The mere fact that we need oxygen to live puts us at a significant risk for oxidative stress. Therefore, the best strategy is to maximize our own body's immune system and antioxidant defenses. This begins by eating a healthy diet. Eating five to seven servings of fruits and vegetables each day (two to three servings of fruits and three to five servings of vegetables) will lower your risk of almost every type of cancer by half. Additionally, we must decrease saturated fat intake and make sure we consume more than 35 grams of fiber each day. We have all heard this before; however, as I will detail in a later chapter, still only nine percent of the population are eating this way.

Medical research is beginning to demonstrate that taking antioxidants in supplementation may be very important in chemoprevention. Supplementation of a good diet over a 20-week period of time with vitamin C, vitamin E, and beta-carotene resulted in a highly significant decrease in oxidative damage to the DNA of both smokers and nonsmokers.[7] Vitamin E has been shown to protect us against exercise-induced DNA damage.[8] Many micronutrients, when taken in supplementation, have been shown to decrease the risk of cancer by protecting the DNA from oxidative damage.

1. Selenium supplementation (200 mcg) has been shown to decrease the risk of prostate cancer by 74 percent, colon cancer by 60 percent, and lung cancer by 30 percent. Many of the antioxidant defense systems are dependent on selenium (especially glutathione) to perform their job in handling free radicals.[9]

2. Folic acid has been shown to protect against the development of precancerous tumors in patients with ulcerative colitis. These patients have a very high risk of developing colon cancer. Diminished folate levels in the body are related to a significantly increased risk of developing several different types of cancer.[10]

3. Vitamins C, E, and A, and provitamin A (beta-carotene) have been shown in several clinical trials to offer protection against developing various types of cancer. Although these studies are not entirely consistent, they support the hypothesis that antioxidant supplementation may decrease the risk of cancer.[11]

4. Animal studies have shown stronger evidence that antioxidant supplements, especially when used in combination, are effective in reducing cancer risk. In one study, vitamin E, vitamin C, beta-carotene, and glutathione significantly inhibited the growth of experimentally induced oral cancers in hamsters. This study demonstrated the strong synergistic effect when these nutrients are used in combination. In other words, the mixture of these antioxidants was much more effective than when these nutrients were used alone.[12]

5. Vitamin E and calcium have been shown to significantly decrease the risk of colon cancer.[13,14]

6. Bioflavonoid antioxidants, which are found in high concentrations in our fruits and vegetables, are known to be potent antioxidants. Clinical studies have shown that they are effective in inhibiting tumor growth and also in decreasing the growth of blood vessels within the tumor itself.[15]

7. CoQ10 has been found to be significantly decreased in patients with cancer. When this nutrient is given to cancer patients in supplementation, not only are their immune systems improved, but also tumor growth is inhibited, and in some cases there is regression.[16]

8. Glutathione has been shown to decrease tumor progression in lung cancer.[17]

CHEMOPREVENTION: PHASE III

Precancerous lesions or growths offer us a unique insight into the use of antioxidants in chemoprevention. In Phase I and Phase II chemoprevention, we were concerned primarily with decreasing the amount of oxidative stress the body had to handle and providing adequate micronutrients to repair any early damage that had been caused to the DNA by oxidative stress. In Phase III, we are concerned about providing adequate nutrients to the cell so it is able to repair significant damage that has occurred to the DNA. It is difficult to follow precancerous tumors within the body, but many studies have been done that follow precancerous tumors that are on the surface of the body. This gives us a window into what may actually happen to these precancerous tumors that are inside our body and not so easy to follow.

These studies primarily look at leukoplakia, which are precancerous tumors found inside the mouths of tobacco chewers, and cervical dysplasia, which are precancerous tumors of the cervix. Both of these are easy to follow since they are on the surface of the body, and their progression or improvement can easily be documented. One hopes that by observing the use of various antioxidants on these tumors, it will give some insight into the possible effect on precancerous tumors within the body. Remember: cancer is a multistage process. Precancerous tumors are quite advanced; the next step is true cancer itself.

There has been great interest in the prevention and treatment of leukoplakia. Leukoplakia are the thickened, white patches that occur along the inside of the mouth in tobacco chewers. It is definitely a precancerous lesion. Several studies have shown that these individuals have low antioxidant levels, and that individuals with the highest level of antioxidants have the lowest risk of developing leukoplakia. Harinder Garewal, MD, wrote a review article on the effect that antioxidants have in the prevention of oral cancer and the reversal of leukoplakia when using antioxidants.[18] There have been several clinical trials which he reviewed:

1. A study in India used vitamin A and beta-carotene. The researchers observed complete remission of the leukoplakia at a rate 10 times greater than the placebo group.
2. A pilot study that used only beta-carotene showed a reversal of leukoplakia back to normal cells in 71 percent of their patients.

3. In an ongoing study in the United States, patients received a combination of beta-carotene, vitamin C, and vitamin E. They saw a response rate of 60 percent.

4. In an ongoing multi-institutional U.S. trial, patients received only beta-carotene and had a response rate of 56 percent.

A study done with male hamsters that had experimentally induced oral cancer looked at using beta-carotene, vitamin E, glutathione, and vitamin C, in combination and alone. There was significant improvement in each group; however, the group receiving the combination had far and away the best results. This was not merely an additional effect but rather a synergistic effect.[19]

Other reviews and studies have shown that the body does have the ability to heal itself if these antioxidant nutrients are provided at optimal levels.[20-22]

Cervical dysplasia is a precancerous lesion of the cervix. Several studies have shown that individuals with low levels of beta-carotene and vitamin C have significantly increased risk of cervical dysplasia. Women with the lowest levels of beta-carotene had two to three times the risk of cervical dysplasia than the women with the highest level of beta-carotene. Women who had an intake of less than 30 mg of vitamin C per day had a ten times greater risk of cervical dysplasia than women who had a vitamin C intake greater than 30 mg per day. Other epidemiological studies have shown dietary deficiencies in vitamin A, vitamin E, beta-carotene, and vitamin C increase the risk of cervical cancer. (23,24)

Beta-carotene supplementation actually has been shown to prevent the progression of cervical dysplasia to cervical cancer. (25) Some clinical trials have shown the role of vitamin C and beta-carotene in reversing or reducing the risk of cervical dysplasia.[19]

There are several ongoing clinical trials that will further determine the roles of antioxidants in reversing precancerous tumors. However, it is simply amazing to me that antioxidants used in supplementation have the ability to reverse these advanced lesions in the majority of patients. This gives us solid evidence that the body has the ability to heal itself when optimal levels of nutrients are provided. These are advanced lesions; the next stage is cancer itself. Since we now realize that cancer is a multistage process that takes decades to develop, what is the potential of reversing these cancerous changes within the cell if we provide these nutrients at a much earlier time? This question has not yet been answered. However, it gives us the basis of using nutritional supplementation throughout a lifetime.

While reviewing the medical literature, my overwhelming conclusion is the fact that the best defense against the development of cancer is our own body. By building up our body's natural antioxidant defense system and immune system, we are giving ourselves the best chance to prevent cancer. I firmly believe that future medical studies will support this conclusion. However, I personally am not going to wait until the evidence is so overwhelming that everyone agrees. It will be too late for me and too late for many of my patients. Nutritional supplementation is relatively inexpensive and safe to be taking over a lifetime. That makes it ideal for chemoprevention.

WHAT IF I ALREADY HAVE CANCER?

Chemoprevention therapies are definitely targeted toward those individuals who have not yet developed cancer. As we have seen throughout this chapter, when a physician diagnoses a cancer, it is in the last stage of a multistage process. There is nothing more difficult than telling your patient that he or she has cancer. Even though cancer treatment has become more effective for some cancers, the overall prognosis is usually not very good. The treatments are harsh and difficult for the patient, causing significant morbidity and even mortality.

Most oncologists and radiation therapists still discourage their patients from taking any kind of nutritional supplementation while they are going through chemotherapy or radiation therapy. Their reasoning is varied and, I feel, reflective of a biased attitude against supplementation in general. I have heard some oncologists actually tell their patients, "Why are you trying to build up your body with nutritional supplementation, when I am trying to tear it down?" Other oncologists are concerned that if patients are taking nutritional supplements that they will be building up the cancer cells antioxidant defenses and will decrease the effectiveness of their chemotherapeutic drugs. Since their drugs work by creating oxidative stress within the body, I can see their reasoning. However, the medical literature does not support their concern. Whenever studies have been done, which look at the use of nutritional supplements in patients who are receiving chemotherapy, the patients using supplements not only tolerate their treatments better, but also have better results from their treatments. Many researchers are now beginning to believe that nutritional supplements actually help protect normal cells and make cancer cells more vulnerable to the chemotherapy.

An early chemotherapuetic drug called methotrexate (which is still used in some cancers and diseases like rheumatoid arthritis) was believed to lose its effectiveness when patients were taking folic acid in supplementation. I feel that this concern with methotrexate has carried over to almost all the other chemotherapeutic drugs. I am personally not aware of any other chemotherapeutic drugs where there is any documented concern in the medical literature about being able to take nutritional supplements with them. In fact, in a 1994 study reported in the Annals of Internal Medicine, patients with rheumatoid arthritis who were taking methotrexate actually tolerated the drug better and had a better response to it if they were taking folic acid in supplementation.

Most of our chemotherapeutic drugs create tremendous amounts of free radicals, thus oxidative stress. This is what is believed to be the mechanism of how these agents destroy or suppress the cancerous tumors. However, the side effects of these drugs are now also being related to this oxidative stress that they cause. The goal of the oncologist is to destroy the cancerous tumors without killing the patient. The treatments not only wipe out the patient's immune system but also may cause devastating damage to other parts of the body. Many patients actually die from the cancer treatments rather than the cancer itself.

There is a basic underlying attitude among physicians who are treating cancer patients. Physicians do not think about it much, but it is there. It is this: We believe the only hope for our patient is our potent drugs. The host (our body) is held in low esteem. We are not concerned with building up our body's natural defenses against the cancer or protecting the body from the devastating side effects of our chemotherapeutic drugs. Our main concern is to make sure the patient survives chemotherapy while we try to arrest the cancer.

The medical literature is beginning to show us a better way of treating our patients with cancer. It is not alternative medicine; it simply involves building up the patient's body (the host) so it can better handle the chemotherapy and/or radiation therapy. The medical literature is beginning to show us that those patients who are taking nutritional supplements while on these treatments actually tolerate their treatments better, and the effectiveness of the chemotherapy is enhanced. The theory behind this approach is to be able to protect our body from the tremendous oxidative stress created by these treatments, while at the same time making these treatments more effective in destroying the cancer cells. Preliminary studies have been encouraging, but more are needed to totally define this issue.[26]

I strongly recommend that my patients who are taking chemotherapy or radiation therapy be on nutritional supplements. If they happen to be taking methotrexate, I do not have them take folic acid the day they take the methotrexate. However, they are encouraged to take their folic acid on all the other days. I believe that within five years everyone will be recommending that their patients who are receiving cancer treatments should also be taking nutritional supplements. Here is just some of the medical evidence to support the use of nutritional supplements in patients who have cancer and are taking cancer treatments:

1. CoQ10 has been shown to stimulate and charge our immune system. There are also several case studies showing that high doses of CoQ10 lead to regression of metastasis in advanced breast cancer. CoQ10 has also been shown to be protective of the heart in patients receiving adriamycin. (Adriamycin is a chemotherapeutic drug that may cause significant damage to the heart as one of its side effects.)[27]

2. A clinical trial using a combination of antioxidants with chemotherapy and radiation therapy in patients with lung cancer showed prolonged survival of these patients. These patients also tolerated their therapy much better. The sooner they started the antioxidants after finding out they had cancer, the better the results.[28]

3. The use of cruciferous antioxidants in patients with breast cancer actually inhibits the growth of these tumors.[29]

4. Antioxidants have been shown to enhance the cytotoxicity of chemotherapeutic drugs used in colon cancer. This means that antioxidants actually improved the effect of these drugs in fighting cancer.[26]

5. Thirty-two typical breast-cancer patients were given a combination of nutritional supplements that were added to the traditional surgical and therapeutic treatment of breast cancer. The nutritional supplementation was vitamin C (2,850 mg), vitamin E (2,500 IU), beta-carotene (32.5 IU), selenium (387 mcg), essential fatty acids, CoQ10, and secondary vitamins and minerals. The main observations of this study were: a) none of the patients died during the period of study (the expected number was four); b) none of the patients showed signs of further metastasis; c) quality of life improved (reduced use of pain killers and no weight loss); and d) six patients showed apparent partial remission.[30]

SUMMARY

Nutritional science offers us the greatest hope in our fight against cancer and several other degenerative diseases. Natural antioxidants and their supporting nutrients are the ideal chemopreventive agents for the following reasons:

1. They are able to limit and even prevent free-radical damage to the DNA nucleus of the cell.
2. They provide the proper nutrients needed for the body to repair any damage that has been previously done.
3. They are safe and may be taken over a lifetime. Pharmaceutical drugs do not share this advantage. Tamoxifen has been shown to decrease the risk of breast cancer; however, its side effects are a great concern.
4. They are inexpensive.
5. Even if you have developed cancer, there is growing evidence that antioxidants will allow you the best defense against the advancement of the disease.
6. They protect your body against the oxidative stress created by the chemotherapy and radiation therapy.
7. They have been shown to augment the cancer-fighting ability of chemotherapy and radiation treatments.
8. They may inhibit the replication and growth of cancer.
9. In some instances, they have been shown to cause tumor regression. Many of the clinical trials regarding chemoprevention of cancer are just beginning. The early studies are encouraging but not conclusive. The next 10 to 20 years will be needed to answer this question more completely, which will be too late to be of any real benefit for most of us. As a clinician, I believe that the evidence is strong enough now to begin recommending the use of nutritional supplements to my patients.

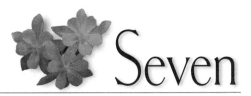 Seven

Oxidative Stress and Your Eyes

The role of oxidative stress as the cause of chronic degenerative diseases involving the eyes has generated significant interest in the use of antioxidant vitamins and minerals as a means to delay, and even prevent, certain diseases of the eye. The main interest is in age-related cataract formation and macular degeneration. There are over 50 million people worldwide who are blind because of cataracts. In the United States, there are more than 1.2 million cataract surgeries performed each year at a cost of over $3.2 billion. Cataract surgery is the most frequently performed surgical procedure in patients over 60 years of age. Its economic impact on the U.S. health care system is substantial. It has been estimated that a 10-year delay in the development of cataracts in the U.S. population would eliminate the need for nearly half of these surgeries. Medical researchers believe it is essential to determine if supplying adequate levels of antioxidant nutrients to the eyes early in life will preserve lens function.

CATARACTS

The function of the lens in the eye is to collect and focus light onto the retina. In order to perform its job properly the lens must remain clear throughout our lifetime. As we age, various components of the lens may be damaged and opacities may occur, leading to senile or age-related cataracts. Research studies support the theory that free oxygen radicals generated by the ultraviolet rays of sunlight and the metabolic activity within the lens of the eye cause cataract formation.[1,2] The lens itself naturally has low levels of antioxidants. Most of the protection against oxidative stress comes from the antioxidants in the fluid and tissues surrounding the lens. Several clinical trials have looked at the possibility that increased dietary and supplemental antioxidants may be protective against this oxidative damage to the lens.

The association between the level of vitamin C, vitamin E, and beta-carotene and the risk of developing cataracts has been demonstrated in several epidemiological studies. In Finland, a case-controlled study showed individuals who had the lowest level of vitamin E and beta-carotene had a four to fivefold increase in the risk of cataract surgery.[3] A recent study found cataract patients had significantly lower levels of vitamin C, vitamin E, and beta-carotene. Those individuals who consumed supplemental vitamins had at least a 50 percent decreased risk of developing cataracts.[4]

There is good medical evidence that the antioxidant protection of young lenses decreases significantly with age. Several different clinical studies are showing a protective effect to the aging eye when patients use various antioxidant supplements. The higher the level of vitamin C in the aqueous fluid around the eye, the greater the protection against cataract formation. Vitamin E and beta-carotene supplements increased the amount of these antioxidants within the tissues in and around the lens. These increased levels of vitamin E and beta-carotene have also been shown to further protect the lens against oxidative damage.[5] Alpha-lipoic acid has been shown to augment the antioxidant effect of all of these antioxidants in protecting the lens of the eye because of its synergistic effect.[6]

There is no doubt in my mind that over the next few years antioxidants will be recommended by all physicians as a way to protect against cataracts. As the clinical trials that are now in progress begin to report their findings, specific levels of antioxidant supplementation will be better known. However, at this time researchers are beginning to agree that supplementation of our diet with antioxidants appears to be useful in the prevention of age-related cataracts.[7]

MACULAR DEGENERATION

In the United States, age-related macular degeneration is the leading cause of blindness in people over 60 years old. Macular degeneration concerns the area of the retina which is responsible for our central vision. It presents in two different forms, dry and wet, both of which affect the macula of the eye. The dry form is characterized by a gradual reduction in central vision, which occurs over a long period of time. However, it may progress to the wet form in about 10 percent of the cases. There is currently no treatment for the dry form of macular degeneration. The wet form causes a more rapid reduction in central vision, the development of new vessels, and possible vessel leakage. The wet form of macular degeneration is being treated at the present time via laser photocoagulation. This treatment, however, does prevent the eventual outcome, which is blindness.

There have been several clinical studies showing that the underlying cause of age-related macular degeneration is free-radical damage to the macula. In the eye, high-energy ultraviolet light and visible blue light create excess free radicals. Studies demonstrate that the eyes' ability to handle these free radicals and to limit the oxidative stress caused by these free radicals deteriorates with age.[8] The Journal of the American Medical Association reported in the November 9, 1994, issue that individuals who have the highest intake of beta-carotene have a 43 percent lower risk of developing macular degeneration compared to those with the lowest level of beta-carotene.[9] Other epidemiological studies have shown that people with macular degeneration had low levels of zinc, selenium, vitamin C, carotenoids, and vitamin E when compared to controls that did not have macular degeneration.[10]

A two-prong attack has been proposed to limit this damage created by free radicals in the hope of preventing, or at least slowing down, the progression of macular degeneration. The first is to shield the eyes against high-energy rays from the sunlight by using high-quality sunglasses. The second is to increase the amount of antioxidants present in the eyes by taking a combination of antioxidants and minerals in supplementation. This will improve the eyes' antioxidant defense system.

In one particular study, 192 patients with macular degeneration were given antioxidants and 61 control patients were untreated. After six months, 87.5 percent of the supplemented patients had visual acuity equal to or better than at the beginning of the study.[11] Only 59 percent of the untreated group had visual acuity equal to or better than at the beginning of the study. A multicenter study that gave a group of patients a specific, 14-component, antioxidant capsule stabilized but did not improve the macular degeneration.[8]

Several studies have identified particular nutrients that appear to be beneficial in macular degeneration. Mixed carotenoids containing lutein and zeaxanthin have been found to improve pigment density in the macula.[13] This offers the macula increased protection against high-energy blue light. They are also both antioxidants which help bring the oxidative stress back into balance. Selenium and zinc supplements have been found to improve our own natural antioxidant defense system (glutathione peroxidase, superoxide dismutase, and catalase).[14] Don't worry about these big names. Just remember: these antioxidant systems need zinc and selenium to do their job. If they are not present in adequate amounts, our defense against free radicals is decreased. Bioflavonoid antioxidants, vitamin C, and vitamin E have also been found to help protect the eye against the development of macular degeneration.[15]

There are many clinical trials that are presently in progress that will help us define specific recommendations for the future. The National Eye Institute is sponsoring a 10-year study called the Age-Related Eye Disease Study involving 4,600 patients. This should clarify some of these issues; unfortunately, the results of these studies will not be available for years.

Eight

Other Degenerative Diseases
Related to Oxidative Stress

There are many other degenerative diseases now being related to oxidative stress. Obviously, coronary artery disease, stroke, and cancer receive the most attention when it comes to research dollars. Recently, however, medical literature has been filled with new evidence that many other diseases are caused by free-radical damage. Alzheimer's dementia, Parkinson's disease, multiple sclerosis, and amyotrophic lateral sclerosis (Lou Gehrig's disease) are some of the neurodegenerative diseases now being tied to oxidative stress.[1] Rheumatoid arthritis, osteoarthritis, and asthma are some other diseases that also may be caused by oxidative stress. These are all devastating, chronic, degenerative diseases that basically have poor medical treatments. Understanding the role of oxidative stress in these diseases will open up several options in hopefully delaying, and even preventing, these diseases.

NEURODEGENERATIVE DISEASES

There are several reasons why the brain and the nerves are vulnerable to oxidative stress:

1. Relative to their size, there is an increased rate of oxidative activity, which creates a significant number of free radicals.
2. There are relatively low levels of antioxidants within the brain and nerve tissue.
3. The central nervous system (the brain) may easily be damaged by oxidative stress, and once damaged it may be dysfunctional for life.[2]

ALZHEIMER'S DEMENTIA

Alzheimer's dementia affects more than two million Americans and is the major cause for admission into nursing homes. Patients not only don't know what day it is, they don't even recognize their own families. There is nothing more devastating than losing our ability to think. Anyone who has had to deal with Alzheimer's dementia within his or her own family understands this tragedy. Quality of life is much more important than length of life, which is why it is so important to protect our health.

Numerous studies have presented evidence that free-radical damage is the cause of Alzheimer's dementia. Recent findings reported by researchers at Case Western Reserve University concluded that increasing oxidative stress with age may account for all aspects of Alzheimer's disease.[3] There is strong evidence that patients with Alzheimer's dementia have significantly depleted levels of antioxidants in their brain and evidence of high levels of oxidative stress. When various antioxidants are given in experimental settings, this oxidative damage is prevented.[4]

There is now great interest in the therapeutic benefits that Alzheimer patients could receive from antioxidants. The New England Journal of Medicine reported in April 1997 a study showing that the progression of Alzheimer's dementia could be significantly slowed by the use of high doses of vitamin E. Patients who were using vitamin E supplements were actually able to remain at home an additional two and one-half to three years longer than the control group.[5] Other clinical trials in which patients who had Alzheimer's dementia used various antioxidants such as vitamin C, vitamin A, vitamin E, zinc, selenium, and rutin (a bioflavonoid antioxidant) have been encouraging.[6]

Several more studies are currently in progress that should reveal much more to us. However, there are basic principles that seem obvious. If antioxidants have this kind of effect on patients with moderately severe Alzheimer's dementia, what would the effect be on those just diagnosed with this disease? Would taking good levels of antioxidant supplements decrease the risk of getting Alzheimer's dementia altogether?

PARKINSON'S DISEASE

A stooped posture, slowness of voluntary movement, rigidity, and a "pill-rolling" tremor characterize Parkinson's disease. A wide variety of studies support the role of free radicals as the underlying cause. There is actual cell death in the area of the brain called the substantia nigra, which leads to decreased production of dopamine. Studies have shown oxidative stress causes this damage. Patients with early Parkinson's disease who received high doses of vitamin C and vitamin E slowed the progression of their disease.[7] Glutathione and N-acetyl L-cysteine were effective in protecting the nerves in the substantia nigra from being destroyed by oxidative stress.[8]

Some studies have not shown improvement of Parkinson's disease with various antioxidants.[9] Several antioxidants have difficulty getting into the tissues around the brain. A drug called selegiline that has an antioxidant effect has been shown to slow the progression of Parkinson's disease.[10] I am amazed that so many studies actually demonstrate a positive effect on a disease process using just a single antioxidant (as explained in detail later, single antioxidants are not effective in handling oxidative stress). With these serious illnesses, the synergistic effect of several different antioxidants, along with their supporting nutrients, is necessary to obtain the best results.

MULTIPLE SCLEROSIS

Multiple sclerosis affects about 250,000 Americans and is about twice as common in women as in men. This disorder affects the myelin sheath (insulation around the nerve). This breakdown of the myelin, called demyelination, results in impairment of the function of the nerve. This is responsible for the clinical symptoms of multiple sclerosis. Dr. LeVine proposed a hypothesis in 1992 that multiple sclerosis was caused by the hydroxyl free radical found in excess within the myelin sheath.[11] Other investigators have documented that oxidative stress was high during active, progressive, multiple sclerosis when compared to those individuals whose multiple sclerosis was in remission or when compared with normal controls.[12] Several other studies have demonstrated strong evidence that the underlying cause of multiple sclerosis is oxidative stress.[13,14,15]

BIONUTRITION

There have not been many clinical trials using antioxidants in patients with multiple sclerosis. However, because of the growing evidence of the involvement of oxidative stress in this disease, there will surely be several clinical trials using antioxidants with these patients in the future. It is interesting to me that the last few treatments released for multiple sclerosis actually build up the immune system. Avonex, betaseron, and immunoglobulins, which have been shown to improve the progression of multiple sclerosis, actually build up our immune system. For years, this disease was treated with immunosuppressive drugs. Most of these treatments did not really show much in the way of improving multiple sclerosis. As you will see in the next chapter, using antioxidant and mineral supplements is a natural way to boost our own immune system. Additionally, these supplements actually increase our ability to handle the underlying oxidative stress.

A REAL-LIFE STORY

A young woman I met a couple of years ago related to me that she had developed multiple sclerosis about 10 years earlier. She had the slowly progressive form of multiple sclerosis, and for six years she had slowly declined. About three years before I met her, she was involved in a double-blind clinical trial for multiple sclerosis using chemotherapy. She had some improvement for the first year, but she went downhill from there. After her last chemotherapy, she was essentially bedridden. She did not know whether she would even be able to walk again. It was at that point that she began an aggressive nutritional supplement program.

She had been on this program for about three months when I had the privilege of meeting her. She was shaking like a leaf but was standing with the help of a cane. Six months later, I was fortunate to see her again, only this time she was able to walk normally and without the use of a cane. During the past year she has had her minor setbacks. However, when I saw her last, she was still able to walk without the use of any aids and was still holding her own. She will be the first to tell you that she still has her multiple sclerosis, but she is in control now.

I have seen actual improvement in individuals with multiple sclerosis several times in the past two years. These individuals are all using high-quality nutritional supplements, along with potent bioflavonoid antioxidants. The body truly possesses the ability to heal itself. Not everyone experiences the kind of results that this young lady did. However, high quality antioxidants, coupled with their supporting nutrients, may offer us the best hope in multiple sclerosis.

AMYOTROPHIC LATERAL SCLEROSIS

Amyotrophic lateral sclerosis (ALS) is better known as Lou Gehrig's disease. Some clinical trials indicate that ALS may be caused by oxidative stress.[16,17] In fact, 20 percent of familial ALS is believed to be caused by a genetic defect in the superoxide dismutase antioxidant defense system. This is a very important internal antioxidant defense system.[18] Other studies show that the underlying nerve damage is caused by excess free radicals. Because of this research, some clinical studies are now being done using a combination of antioxidants as part of the treatment.[19,20] One of these studies on 36 ALS patients showed an increase in survival of six months. This may not seem like much, but it is a step in the right direction. By way of comparison, the only drug approved for ALS by the FDA showed an average increase in survival of three months at a cost of about $700 per month.

My personal experience has shown me that in order to have any hope of altering the course of such a severe disease as ALS, you need to be very aggressive. Studies must look at high doses of several antioxidants used in combination. The studies should look into the more potent bioflavonoid antioxidants, such as proanthocyanidins. This category of antioxidants has been studied almost exclusively in Europe. They have been found to be 50 times more potent than vitamin E and 20 times more potent than vitamin C in their ability to handle oxidative stress. In fact, proanthocyanidins are the most potent natural antioxidants that have been discovered to date. They have an important role in neurodegenerative diseases because they readily cross over into the fluid around the brain and nerves. Most antioxidants have difficulty doing this. These bioflavonoids will make great optimizers, which I believe should be added to combinations of the more common antioxidants. I have seen significant results in patients who are using this approach.

INFLAMMATORY BOWEL DISEASE

Crohn's disease and ulcerative colitis are inflammatory diseases of the small and large intestines. Several clinical trials show that both of these diseases are caused, at least in part, by oxidative stress.[21-25] The inflammatory process in the mucosa of the bowel creates a significant increase in free radicals. This places a tremendous burden on the antioxidant defense system of the bowel. Several clinical trials have demonstrated a marked depletion in the antioxidant nutrients within the mucosa of patients with these diseases.[26-29]

BIONUTRITION

Since these diseases affect the bowels, there is a good possibility that the bowels are not absorbing the necessary nutrients they need from their food. This makes it even more critical that these patients be taking nutritional supplements in order to build up their depleted antioxidant defense system.

PULMONARY DISEASE

There have been consistent findings in patients with chronic obstructive lung disease (emphysema) and asthma. The lungs are exposed to more pollutants than almost any part of our body. Not only do we see the air we breathe, we can now taste it. Air pollution contains ozone, nitrogen dioxide, sulfur dioxide, and several different hydrocarbons. All of these pollutants significantly increase the amount of free radicals present within the lining of the lung and have been related to emphysema and asthma.[30] Studies have shown that in the acute phases of both these diseases, oxidative stress is high. Antioxidant defense systems are soon depleted.[31] Vitamin C is one of the most important antioxidants in the lung since most of this attack takes place in the aqueous fluid within the lung tissue itself. Vitamin C levels, along with other antioxidants, have been found to be depleted during these acute attacks. Epidemiological studies have shown that low dietary intake of vitamin C significantly increases your risk of developing asthma.[32]

We have discussed the fact that cigarette smoke is the greatest cause of oxidative stress in the lungs and throughout the body. Studies involving smokers have shown an overwhelming imbalance of oxidants (free radicals) over antioxidants. This oxidant- to-antioxidant imbalance can lead to lung injury due to direct, unprotected, oxidative damage to the surface cells of the lung. Connective lung tissue is also damaged. This is the obvious cause of chronic obstructive lung disease (emphysema) in smokers.

These studies show an impressive imbalance in the level of free radicals, compared to the level of antioxidants in patients with asthma and chronic obstructive lung disease. This is especially apparent in acute flareups.[33] These findings strongly suggest that we should perform interventional trials with supplemental antioxidants to enhance our antioxidant defenses in asthma and chronic obstructive lung disease. This is the best way to bring the oxidant/antioxidant imbalance back in line. Remember: balance is the key. If we are going to be out of balance, we will need to have greater amount of antioxidants than oxidants.

ARTHRITIS

Arthritis is a degenerative process of the joints. It doesn't usually shorten lives, but it causes significant pain and disability. There has been great interest among researchers for the past 20 years into the role of oxidative stress in arthritis. Most of the studies have not distinguished between rheumatoid arthritis and osteoarthritis (degenerative arthritis) when looking at free-radical reactions and these diseases. Henrotin wrote a very comprehensive review article in 1992 in regards to oxidative stress and its involvement in inflammatory joint disease.[34] Several recent studies have also established the possible cause of these diseases to be the result of oxidative stress.[35]

When researchers analyzed joint fluid from an inflamed joint, they noted a significant increase in the number of free radicals,[36] while fluid from a normal joint contains absolutely no free radicals. Studies have shown a significant increase in risk for developing rheumatoid arthritis in individuals who have low levels of vitamin E, beta-carotene, and selenium.[37] Other studies have shown that low levels of vitamins C and D are found in patients who have more severe joint disease which is progressing rapidly.[38]

There are many separate factors that may cause an increase of oxidative stress within inflamed joints. These joints have a significant inflammatory response within the joint space, especially in rheumatoid arthritis. Neutrophils (a type of white cell) are a predominant cell in this inflammatory response. They have been shown to release a significant amount of free radicals within the joint space. This causes a significant rise in oxidative stress. When we exercise an inflamed joint, there is a lack of oxygen to parts of the joint space. Once we quit exercising, the tissues again receive oxygen. During this reperfusion phase, studies have shown a significant rise in free-radical production. Certain cells from the cartilage called chondrocytes in an inflamed joint also have been found to actively generate free radicals. These different sources of increased free-radical production within the inflamed joint cause significant oxidative stress. This overloads the antioxidant defense system of the joint space. The synovial fluid (joint fluid), which is usually very thick, becomes thin. The cartilage is damaged within this environment. Therefore, the process of joint destruction takes place.[39]

Current studies are using antioxidant micronutrients as part of the therapy for patients with either rheumatoid or osteoarthritis. One study concluded that a high intake of antioxidant micronutrients (especially vitamin C) reduced the risk of cartilage loss and disease progression in people with osteoarthritis.[40] There have been studies with superoxide dismutase (SOD), an internal antioxidant that has significantly slowed down the progression of rheumatoid arthritis.[41] Although the results were not consistent with vitamin E, several studies showed significant improvement in the symptoms of arthritis.[42] Supplementation with 160 mcg of selenium resulted in significant improvement in 40 percent of patients with rheumatoid arthritis.[43]

A REAL-LIFE STORY

One of my patients developed rheumatoid arthritis, which was documented by a rheumatologist. He had significant pain and swelling of his joints in his feet and hands. He was unable to wear his shoes or even make a fist with either hand. He had tried several different nonsteroidal anti-inflammatories, but with no improvement. The rheumatologist wanted to place him on methotrexate, which is one of the chemotherapeutic drugs used for rheumatoid arthritis. I encouraged my patient to try this drug because nothing had helped and his disease was progressing rapidly. He wanted to wait, however, as he was worried about the potential side effects.

He started on a complete, balanced, nutritional program that I was using in my practice. During the first six months he did not show any significant improvement. At that time, he still did not want to try methotrexate. We increased some of the more potent antioxidants he was taking, while maintaining the basic antioxidant and mineral supplements. He began to show significant improvement within three weeks. He came into my office wearing shoes instead of slippers for the first time in two years. Within the next month he was able to start making a fist. Now, he not only has absolutely no pain or swelling in his feet and hands but is able to make a tight fist. He was even able to mow his lawn, something he thought he would never be able to do again.

Some physicians will say this is a coincidence – the patient merely went into remission, which can happen in rheumatoid arthritis. This may be true. The patient, however, could care less what is true. He has continued to do great for the past two years after struggling with his rheumatoid arthritis for years.

CLINICAL APPLICATIONS

In this chapter, we have mentioned a few of the several diseases now being investigated. Further studies are needed to define the true role of oxidative stress in these diseases. Clinical trials are needed to define the effectiveness of antioxidants as an addition to traditional therapies. Many of these preliminary studies demonstrate the devastating effect of having more free radicals than antioxidants. While medical research is determining the role of antioxidants in these diseases, common sense tells me that building the body's antioxidant defense system by taking nutritional supplements is wise. The level of nutritional supplements I use in my practice is safe, and the results have been encouraging. Remember: we are building the body's natural defense against oxidative stress. We are merely bringing the basic cause of these diseases (oxidative stress) under better control.

Nine

Antioxidants and the Immune System

The immune system is our personal police force that is working against any foreign invader and is definitely one of our greatest defenses against disease. Bionutrition means providing all of the proper nutrients to the body at optimal levels so that our immune system may function at its peak level. In this chapter we will learn how antioxidants and their supporting micronutrients build our immune system.

Physicians over the years have developed an attack philosophy when it comes to the treatment of disease. I believe this stems from physicians' success in the treatment of infectious disease with antiobiotics starting in the middle of this century. This approach has carried over into our treatment of chronic degenerative diseases today. We attack many of these chronic diseases with aggressive medical and surgical therapies, but these therapies are in total disregard of the host, which is our own body.

In the case of autoimmune diseases, I was always taught that they were the result of an overreactive immune system. This was because in these diseases our immune system was now attacking our own body; in other words, we are attacking ourself instead of a foreign invader. If our body attacks the joints, we have rheumatoid arthritis. If it attacks the myelin sheath of the nerve, we have multiple sclerosis. If it attacks our bowels, we have ulcerative colitis or Crohn's disease.

Most of the actual damage to the body seen in these autoimmune diseases is caused by oxidative stress. But now that I have had such success with building my patient's immune system using micronutrients, I believe that these diseases are not so much the result of an overreactive immune system as they are the result of a confused immune system. As we build up the immune system in these patients using antioxidants and their supporting micronutrients, the immune system becomes less confused and actually begins to recognize the self again. So, in this chapter you will begin to realize that nutritional supplements not only improve our own antioxidant defense system but also our body's immune system.

Malnutrition is the most common cause of a depressed immune system. There is a consensus among experts in this field that micronutrient intake is one of the most important aspects of host defense.

As a physician, would you rather treat a patient with a healthy or an unhealthy immune system? Without a healthy host (our body), drugs are not very effective. Consider the case of treating a serious infection in a patient with full-blown AIDS or a patient whose immune system has been wiped out with chemotherapuetic drugs. You may use the most potent antibiotics in the world and still not be able to help your patient survive. However, when we use our medications in patients with a healthy immune system, they can be very effective. We must always remember that a competent immune system is the physician's greatest ally.

Adequate host defense activity critically depends upon the micronutrient status of the individual. The most important factor is the cellular oxidant/antioxidant balance. Free radicals are used by the immune system to help destroy viruses and bacteria. That's right – not all free radicals are bad. However, the antioxidant status must be at its peak to help protect our own cells as we destroy these invaders. Whether it is a bacteria, a virus, or a foreign body, a healthy immune system is able to handle the situation. There are natural killer cells produced by the immune system which also are able to attack tumor cells. Our immune system is critical in tumor surveillance.

Despite the introduction of antibiotics in the war against infectious disease, the nutritional status of an individual is still the most important factor in host resistance to infection. Malnutrition is the most common cause of a depressed immune system. There is a consensus among experts in this field that micronutrient intake is one of the most important aspects of host defense.

MICRONUTRIENTS AND THE IMMUNE SYSTEM

Vitamin E plays an important role in building the immune system as the principal fat-soluble antioxidant. Since vitamin E is incorporated within the cell membranes of white cells, it is able to interact with the excess free radicals produced during this immune response. Studies have demonstrated that when there are adequate stores of vitamin E, not only are certain white cells increased but their longevity is increased.[1] R. P. Tengerdy was able to show clearance of E. coli from the blood after an experimental infection was significantly improved when there was an optimal supply of vitamin E, as compared to controls who were not supplemented with vitamin E. He also observed that the mortality rate from this infection was significantly reduced.[2] These same findings were noted in several other infections. This enhancement of the immune system with vitamin E supplementation has been well established in medical literature.

Clinical studies have also demonstrated that this immune-enhancing effect of vitamin E supplementation was even greater in the elderly and in individuals who had malabsorption syndromes.[3] Vitamin E supplementation can also protect against the immunosuppressive effects of cortisol in the course of stress reactions.[4]

When beta-carotene was taken in supplementation, there was a significant increase in the number of circulating T-helper cells, a type of white cell. Also noted was a significant increase in natural killer cells, which constitute an important part of our defense system against tumor cells.[5] This greatly improves the tumor surveillance of our immune system.[6]

Linus Pauling has been influential in making everyone aware of the importance of supplemental vitamin C and its ability to enhance the immune system. Although we are still arguing whether massive doses of vitamin C can actually prevent the common cold, almost everyone agrees that it is able to reduce the severity and length of the cold. Vitamin C has been shown to improve the function of the phagocytes (Pac-Man-like white cells).[7] This significantly improves the first line of defense against bacterial infections. There is more wisdom in taking good daily doses of vitamin C than in massive doses just when you think you are coming down with an infection. Supplementation with one gram of vitamin C daily for more than two months showed a striking enhancement of several aspects of the immune system (IgA, IgM, and C3 complement production).[8] Vitamin C also has the ability to regenerate vitamin E and handle excess free radicals within the plasma. Both of these properties further enhance vitamin C's ability to improve the immune system.

Another important player in enhancing the immune system is the most important intracellular antioxidant, glutathione. Elevation of glutathione levels within the cell by either supplementation of glutathione or by giving its precursor, N-acetyl L-cysteine, significantly enhances the immune response of lymphocytes (a type of white cell).[9] This effect has also been confirmed in patients with full-blown AIDS who are significantly deficient in T-helper lymphocytes.[10]

Zinc is needed in almost every aspect of the immune system. When there is a deficient amount of available zinc, there is a significant suppression of several aspects of the immune system.[11] When there are very low levels of zinc, the number of lymphocytes decreases and the function of many white cells is severely reduced. There are also lower levels of thymic hormone, which is a strong stimulus of the immune system.[12] All of these effects are reversed with zinc supplementation. Many people reach for their zinc-containing lozenges whenever they get a cold. Studies have shown that taking these lozenges every two hours can shorten the length of a cold by several days. Researchers believe that the zinc not only boosts the immune system but also inhibits the replication of the virus.[13]

A word of caution is necessary here: If this high dose of zinc is taken for too long, it can actually suppress the immune system. I am not against short-term use of high doses of zinc or even vitamin C with colds; however, consistent, long-term use of good doses of these two nutrients in supplementation is better for the antioxidant defense system and the immune system.[14]

CoQ10 taken in supplementation significantly increased the levels of some immunoglobulins, along with enhancing the effect of the macrophages (a type of white cell.)[15] Certain bioflavonoids and other potent antioxidants have been shown to have an effect on improving the immune system. Their specific effect needs to be established in further clinical studies.

As we age, there is generally an association between an impaired immune system and increased frequency of infection. This is a major cause of illness and the fourth most common cause of death in the elderly. Clinical trials that give the elderly nutritional supplements have shown a significant improvement in their immune systems.[16] This generally requires supplementing these patients for a full year before the maximum effect is realized. (To build up the immune system in younger patients requires more than six months of nutritional supplementation.) Elderly patients so supplemented had significantly less frequent infection-related illnesses. These trials have shown the prevalence of micronutrient deficiencies in apparently healthy elderly individuals. In fact, researchers have concluded that the first sign of these micronutrient deficiencies may be a depressed immune system. There is solid evidence that elderly patients simply cannot absorb the nutrients as well from their foods. However, supplementation with antioxidants and minerals is effective in not only improving their antioxidant defense system but also in enhancing their immune system.

Remember: supplementation with micronutrients has been shown in medical literature to significantly improve our immune system, whether we are young or old. Children's immune function actually responds very well to supplementation. Just remember, it takes six to twelve months to realize the full benefit.

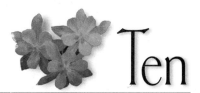

Ten

CHAPTER

Diabetes Mellitus

Diabetes has become epidemic in the United States and in many industrialized nations in the world. In my clinical practice, I have observed a troubling pattern. Many patients, beginning in their late thirties or early forties, start gaining a significant amount of weight. Then they start to develop increased levels of cholesterol and triglycerides. Shortly thereafter, they begin to develop hypertension, which must be treated. By their late forties, they become diabetic. Some refer to this as syndrome X. I observe this scenario over and over in my practice. The sad thing is that I know my patients are now aging much faster than they need to or should be. They are actually giving up 10 to 15 years of life expectancy.

Diabetes has increased more than five times in the past 35 years. There are more than eight million people in the United States who have been diagnosed with diabetes; 95 percent of these have developed it as an adult (adult-onset diabetes mellitus, or as it is now called, type II diabetes). There are estimated to be eight million people in the United States who have diabetes but have not been diagnosed. However, the most concerning statistic is the fact that there are more

℘

BIONUTRITION

than 23 million Americans that have preclinical diabetes or impaired glucose tolerance. Diabetes has been estimated to cost $150 billion a year in the United States – 15 percent of health care costs.

This tremendous cost of diabetes is related to both short- and long-term complications. Although there has been great progress in handling short-term complications, there has been poor progress in dealing with long-term complications. Diabetes is now the leading cause of new cases of blindness in the United States because of diabetic retinopathy.[1]

Diabetes is responsible for over one-third of the new cases of end-stage renal disease in this country.[2] Premature heart attacks, peripheral vascular disease (loss of limb), and stroke are very high in diabetics, in spite of traditional medical treatments.

As we studied the risk of hardening of the arteries in Chapter 3, we looked at the culprit being oxidized LDL and not native LDL. In diabetics, oxidized LDL actually becomes glycosalated (filled with sugar) because of the increased level of sugar in the blood. Studies have shown that this glycosalated, oxidized LDL is even more prone to cause hardening of the arteries than just simply oxidized LDL.[3]

DR. STRAND'S THEORY OF THE EVOLUTION OF DIABETES

Diabetes mellitus does not just start one day. It is a progression of several events that occur over a 10-to-15-year period. Americans believe that a high-carbohydrate, low-fat diet is the healthiest way to eat. Dieticians believe a carbohydrate is a carbohydrate, with absolutely no distinction as to how fast we absorb the sugar from that carbohydrate. However, carbohydrates are simply long chains of sugars that are released at various rates in the body. This has been documented in the medical literature as glycemic index (the rate at which sugars are released from the carbohydrate into the bloodstream). Carbohydrates such as white bread, white flour, pasta, white rice, and potatoes release their sugars rapidly (high-glycemic foods) and in some studies as fast as if you were simply eating refined sugar. Foods such as green beans, rye bread, whole apples, and cauliflower release their sugars slowly (low-glycemic foods). The rapid rise in blood sugar after a high-glycemic meal stimulates the release of insulin from the pancreas to control the blood sugar level. This type of diet stimulates the release of insulin over and over, day after day. It is a lot like crying "wolf" all the time. Eventually, we are not going to be as sensitive to our insulin as we once were. We then develop insulin resistance.

Insulin resistance is the beginning event of a complicated metabolic change that occurs in our body. First, we fall into this preclinical diabetic state; we have impaired glucose tolerance, but we are not diabetic. Elevated cholesterol and triglycerides soon follow. Shortly thereafter, we develop hypertension. Then, a few years later, we actually become diabetic.

In a six-year Nurses Health study of 65,000 women whose diets were high in carbohydrates from white bread, potatoes, white rice, and pasta (high-glycemic diet), participants had two and one-half times the risk of developing type II (adult onset) diabetes than those who ate a low-glycemic diet. The researchers excluded other risk factors such as weight, exercise level, and family history. The increased risk was related strictly to diet.

In the newly diagnosed diabetic patient, clinical studies have shown that as many as 60 percent of our patients already have significant cardiovascular disease. This means that the vascular disease has progressed significantly before we even have a chance to treat the patient. We are essentially behind the eight ball before we even get started.

Walter Willett, a professor of epidemiology and nutrition at the Harvard School of Public Health and a co-author of this study, found the results of this study, along with other studies, so convincing that he recommended that the government change the Food Guide Pyramid. The Food Guide Pyramid recommends six to eleven servings of carbohydrates a day but does not make any distinction whether these are high-glycemic or low-glycemic carbohydrates. He believes that white bread, potatoes, white rice, and pasta should actually be moved up the Food Guide Pyramid and considered in the Sweets category because metabolically they are the same. I couldn't agree more.

VASCULAR RISK OF TYPE II DIABETES

Why are we not very effective in preventing vascular disease in our diabetic patients? It is primarily because of the length of time that transpires before an actual diagnosis of diabetes is made. In the newly diagnosed diabetic patient, clinical studies have shown that as many as 60 percent of our patients already have significant cardiovascular disease.[4] This means that the vascular disease has progressed significantly before we even have a chance to treat the patient. We are essentially behind the eight ball before we even get started.

Physicians must go back and rethink this whole problem if we are going to have any hope of changing this tremendous health risk. Most diabetic patients have had their diabetes for eight to ten years before they were actually diagnosed. Because of this fact, the American Diabetic Association has now defined diabetes to be present in a patient if their fasting blood sugar level is over 125. This will definitely allow us to begin treating our diabetic patients sooner. However, there are other facts we must consider in order to help our patients even more.

ANOTHER REASON WE NEED TO TAKE SUPPLEMENTS

Clinical trials have demonstrated that patients with preclinical diabetes or impaired glucose tolerance have significantly lower levels of antioxidants.[5] There was evidence of significantly increased levels of oxidative stress, while at the same time noting a depletion of our antioxidant defense system. In other trials, this oxidative stress was more significant in those who had secondary complications of their diabetes like retinopathy or cardiovascular disease.[6] These authors felt that antioxidant supplementation should be added to the traditional insulin treatment as a means to help arrest these complications. The Neurology Department at the Mayo Clinic reported a study where they experimentally created diabetic peripheral neuropathy. They concluded that this complication was indeed caused by oxidative stress. They were able to reverse this nerve damage by giving alpha-lipoic acid, which is both a fat-soluble and water-soluble antioxidant. They also noted that if the subjects had good levels of alpha-lipoic acid because of supplementation before the researchers induced the oxidative stress, there was no nerve damage.[7]

There are many micronutrients that have been found to be deficient in patients with preclinical and frank diabetes. One of the most important is chromium. Chromium is critical in the metabolism of glucose and the action of insulin. There are studies that show that almost 90 percent of the American population are deficient in chromium.[8] Chromium has been shown to greatly improve our insulin sensitivity, especially in those who are chromium deficient.[9]

Vitamin E not only improves antioxidant defenses but also has been shown to improve insulin resistance.[10] In other studies, a low vitamin E level has been an independent and strong predictor for the development of adult-onset diabetes mellitus. There was a five-fold increase in the risk of developing diabetes in those individuals who had low levels of vitamin E.[11]

Magnesium deficiency has been associated with both type I and II diabetes.[12]

This low level of magnesium has also been associated with an increased risk of diabetic patients developing diabetic retinopathy.[13] When this deficiency is corrected in the elderly, there is a significant improvement in the function of insulin. Diagnosing magnesium deficiency is very difficult. We use serum magnesium levels where only 0.3 percent of the body's total magnesium is located. Cellular levels of magnesium are much more sensitive and accurate. Magnesium deficiency may be the most underdiagnosed electrolyte abnormality today.[14]

CLINICAL APPLICATION

Most of this information is just now evolving. My goal as a practicing clinician, however, is not only to prevent the complications of diabetes but diabetes itself. Since insulin resistance and oxidative stress seem to be the initial problems, these need to be addressed. The mainstay of diabetic prevention and treatment will always be a good healthy diet and moderate exercise. Both of these modalities increase insulin sensitivity and decrease diabetic complications. However, I believe there is enough evidence at this time to recommend the addition of nutritional supplements to all of my patients, whether they have diabetes or not. It is often years before the patient actually realizes that he or she has become diabetic. The damage is already occurring, but we are just not aware of it. As with heart disease and cancer, we need to do whatever is possible to prevent diabetes. Following a well-balanced, nutritional supplement program while you are still healthy, I believe, will significantly decrease your risk of developing diabetes. If you are diabetic, the need for antioxidant supplementation is even more critical for you to help avoid the devastating complications of your diabetes.

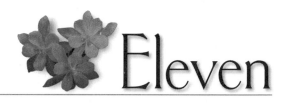

Eleven

Osteoporosis

O steoporosis is an epidemic nutritional deficiency in the United States. There are more than 25 million Americans who have osteoporosis, and the cost to the economy of the United States is about $14 billion annually. At least 1.2 million fractures occur each year in the United States as a direct result of osteoporosis. I have had patients fracture a hip as they simply walked into my office – without any kind of fall or injury. Spontaneous compression fractures of the vertebrae in the back cause tremendous pain and suffering in my patients with osteoporosis.

It is sometimes forgotten that bone is active, living tissue continually remodeling itself through osteoblastic (bone forming) and osteoclastic (bone resorbing) activity. It is constantly engaged in biochemical reactions which are dependent on many different micronutrients and enzyme systems. Therefore, like any living tissue, bone has diverse nutritional needs. It is not just a collection of calcium crystals. The American diet, with its high intake of white breads, white flour, refined sugars, and fat, has been shown to be deficient in many of the essential nutrients that bone needs. Inadequate intake of any of these nutrients required for healthy bone could help lead to osteoporosis. All of these nutrients must be present at optimal levels if we are going to have any effect on decreasing the amount of osteoporosis in this country.

In order to reduce the risk of fractures of the spine, hip, and wrist, we must pay attention to several factors:

1. Preserving adequate bone mass.
2. Preventing the loss of the protein matrix.
3. Making sure that bone has all the proper nutrients it needs to repair and replace damaged areas.

CALCIUM

There is no doubt that calcium deficiency can lead to osteoporosis. However, studies have shown that skeletal calcium depletion was present in only 25 percent of postmenopausal women. Calcium supplements in these women were found to increase bone mass; however, the supplements had no effect on the other 75 percent who were not calcium deficient.[3] Recent studies of calcium and vitamin D supplementation have shown a slowing down of osteoporosis but not the prevention of it. These studies have also shown a reduction in fractures of the hip, spine, and wrist.[4]

Calcium is an essential nutrient in the fight against osteoporosis. Calcium should be taken in supplementation at a level of 800 to 1,500 mg daily. Children also need this level of supplementation. In fact, studies show that children given this level of calcium prior to puberty will increase their bone density by nearly five percent.[5] This increase in bone-density level will be carried with them throughout their lifetime.

MAGNESIUM

Magnesium has many important functions throughout the body, including maintaining the electrical conduction of the heart. Magnesium is also important in several biochemical reactions that take place within bone. Alkaline phosphatase, an enzyme required in the process of forming new bone crystals, is activated by magnesium. Vitamin D needs magnesium to convert it to its most active form. If there is a depletion in magnesium, this can lead to a syndrome of vitamin D resistance.[8]

Dietary surveys have shown 80 to 85 percent of American women consume a magnesium-deficient diet.

VITAMIN K

Vitamin K is required to synthesize osteocalcin, a protein found in large amounts within bone.[9] It is therefore critical in bone formation, remodeling, and repair. In a series of 16 patients with osteoporosis, it was found that the vitamin K concentration was only 35 percent of that in the control subjects.[10] In a clinical trial, supplementing vitamin K in patients with osteoporosis reduced urinary calcium loss by 18 to 50 percent.[11] The clinical evidence shows that in patients who have osteoporosis the need for vitamin K is much greater.

VITAMIN D

Vitamin D is absolutely necessary if we are to have any chance of absorbing any calcium from our diet. A recent study in the New England Journal of Medicine showed that 93 percent of the acutely ill medical patients entering Massachusetts General Hospital were deficient in vitamin D. Even though vitamin D is produced in the skin when it is exposed to sunlight, as patients age they spend less and less time out in the sun. Hence, vitamin D deficiencies become very common. Vitamin D taken orally must be converted to its biologically active form, vitamin D3. Impaired conversion of vitamin D to its active form may be more of a problem than deficient intake. This gives rationale to the supplementation of vitamin D by in its active form, vitamin D3.

Studies show that patients with osteoporosis treated with vitamin D3 increased calcium absorption and reduced bone loss.[12]

MANGANESE

Manganese is necessary for the synthesis of connective tissue in cartilage and bone.[13] Like magnesium, manganese is lost in the processing of whole grains into refined flour. A study of osteoporotic women showed that their manganese level was only 25 percent that of the controls.[14]

FOLIC ACID, VITAMIN B6, AND VITAMIN B12

Does this combination sound familiar? It should. Homocysteine is not only bad for your blood vessels, but it is also bad for your bones. Individuals with severe elevations of homocysteine have been found to have significant osteoporosis.[15] An interesting point about homocysteine, which was not made earlier, is the fact that premenopausal women have great efficiency in breaking down methionine and not having a buildup of homocysteine. This changes dramatically after menopause. Postmenopausal women have much higher levels of homocysteine.

Could this, in part, explain both the increased risks of heart disease and osteo-porosis in postmenopausal women? The fact remains that these women need higher amounts of folic acid, vitamin B6, and vitamin B12.

BORON

Boron has become an interesting nutrient when it comes to bone metabolism. When boron is given in supplementation, the urinary excretion of calcium decreases by 40 percent.[16] Also, there is a significant increase in 17 beta-estradi-ol, which is the most biologically active form of human estrogen.[17] This is not believed to increase the risk of cancer. The cancer-causing effect of estrogen is dose related; the amount of estrogen effect produced by boron equals only five percent of the oral dose. Supplementation with 3 mg of boron is more than adequate.

SILICON

Silicon is important in its ability to strengthen the connective-tissue matrix by cross-linking collagen strands. Patients with osteoporosis, where the generation of new bone is desirable, need increased amounts of silicon.[18]

ZINC

This mineral is essential for the normal functioning of vitamin D. Low serum zinc levels were found in the serum and bones of patients with osteoporosis. [19]

It is clear that osteoporosis is not simply a calcium and estrogen problem. When you supply all of the nutrients needed for bone metabolism, you give yourself a greater chance of avoiding osteoporosis. Estrogen therapy is a decision you and your physician must make.

Osteoporosis has been presented to the public as a disease merely dependent on estrogen and calcium. However, it is important to remember that estrogen slows the loss of bone but does not prevent it.[1] There is growing concern over the possible increased risk of breast cancer in women who are on estrogen replacement. In 1997, the New England Journal of Medicine reported that a study of women who were on estrogen replacement for more than five years had over a 40 percent increased risk in developing breast cancer when compared to those women who did not take estrogen replacement.[2] This is very concerning to me. Why should physicians be placing their patients on routine estrogen replace-ment when they know they are significantly increasing their patients' risk of breast cancer? Physicians justify these treatments by saying that good of estrogen replacement outweighs the bad. Estrogen replacement decreases the risk of heart disease, possibly decreasing the risk of Alzheimer's dementia, and it decreases the risk of osteoporosis, while at the same time decreasing the patient's symptoms of menopause.

I believe there are better ways to decrease these risks, while at the same time not increasing the risk of breast cancer. In my office, we not only recommend the use of natural progesterone (in either the cream or micronized tablet form), but also on occasion we will use low levels of natural estrogen if necessary. We also encourage the use of natural phytoestrogens. When we combine these recommendations with a high-quality, nutritional supplement program, we have actually seen an increase in bone density on Dexa scans in several of our patients. We also lower the risk of heart disease, and I believe Alzheimer's dementia, and our patients usually are able to control their menopausal symptoms.

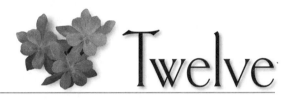

Twelve

Fibromyalgia

My wife has fibromyalgia. Living with this illness for 15 years has totally changed my perception of the seriousness of this disease and, in turn, chronic fatigue syndrome. For most of the time that she has had fibromyalgia, my wife has needed to be in bed by at least 8 P.M., only to arise at 7 A.M. just as tired as when she went to sleep. She suffered from early morning stiffness. The mental fog, muscle spasms (my massage technique certainly improved), fatigue, and pain were daily encounters with which she had to learn to live. My wife always joked that she thought marrying a physician would allow her to improve her health. I am afraid I was not the answer.

Three years ago my wife developed a very serious pneumonia that resolved very slowly. When the pneumonia finally did clear, she developed severe fatigue, which persisted for well over three months. During this time, she was unable to be up for more than two hours at a time. She developed severe asthma. She was placed on bursts of steroids, nebulizer treatments, and biaxin (an antibiotic) by her pulmonologist. She was also under the care of an infectious disease specialist.

They both were doing everything possible. Neither was very optimistic about any significant improvement in my wife's condition in the near future.

The frustration that I felt as a physician who was really unable to do anything for his wife was tremendous. I now realize the frustration that patients with fibromyalgia have with their doctors. Since there is only symptomatic treatment for chronic fatigue syndrome and fibromyalgia, it is truly frustrating for both physician and patient.

When my wife was struggling with one of her most difficult times, she asked if she could try some nutritional supplements given to her by a friend. For 23 years, I had done pretty much everything to discourage my patients from taking any kind of supplements. However, my response to her request even shocked me. I told her she could try anything since it was obvious that the medical profession did not have the answers to her present problems.

Within a week she was better. Within three weeks she was back to her normal self and actually off all of her medications. Over the next year she not only totally recovered, but she had more energy than she had had in years. She has recovered three to four hours of each day of her life. She now only sleeps six or seven hours each night. She has significantly less pain and fewer muscle spasms, and her energy level has surpassed mine.

Obviously, this entire episode caused me to take a long, hard look at my bias against nutritional supplements. This book is the outcome of my research through current medical literature which followed my wife's dramatic improvement. Her recovery challenged me to try to understand what had happened. This was the beginning of my newfound interest in nutritional supplements.

Shortly after this experience, I read a book by Kenneth Cooper, MD, called The Antioxidant Revolution. I have always admired Dr. Cooper, who started the exercise revolution back in the early 1970s. I actually became so intrigued with his book that I researched his research. One part of the book truly caught my attention. At his aerobics clinic in Dallas, Dr. Cooper evaluated several athletes suffering from an overtraining syndrome. There, at his aerobic center, he demonstrated that oxidative stress was the cause of this syndrome. When people exercise mildly or moderately, the body is usually able to handle the amount of free radicals that are produced. However, when the amount of exercise an individual does is excessive, the amount of free radicals the body produces goes up exponentially – literally, off the chart. It struck me that these athletes with this overtraining syndrome had the same symptoms as patients with chronic fatigue syndrome and fibromyalgia. Could it be possible that the root cause of chronic fatigue and immune dysfunction syndrome is oxidative stress?

As we learn more and more about how oxidative stress can cause degenerative diseases, one has to wonder if this is the cause of the chronic fatigue/fibromyalgia syndromes. These syndromes are not high on the totem pole for research dollars. I have been unable to find any studies that have even looked at this as a possibility. I am hopeful that more funds will be allocated toward these very serious, disabling diseases.

Many patients arrive at my office with the simple complaint of fatigue of a few months duration. Since physicians are disease-oriented, we set out trying to find a cause of this fatigue. Most of the time we are not able to find a disease process that explains the patient's complaints. I used to send these people out the door after I told them there was nothing wrong. I am sure they believed I was really saying that everything was just in their head. Now, I believe that this is the beginning of oxidative stress, and I label these patients as being immunologically depressed. If they are allowed to go untreated, some will slowly recover but many will become worse and either fall into chronic fatigue syndrome or fibromyalgia syndrome. Usually, these patients will grind along until they have a severe illness, injury, or stressful situation, which many times sets off these two illnesses. All of these situations cause significant increases in oxidative stress, which the body must try to handle. I believe that both of these syndromes have the same cause (oxidative stress) but with differing expressions when it comes to the way it affects us.

For the past three years, I have been evaluating and treating this group of patients with the belief that the underlying cause is oxidative stress. Since these diseases are able to mimic many other diseases, I must first rule out any other possible disease. I then place these patients on a complete, balanced, nutritional supplement program with the addition of higher doses of proanthocyanidins and CoQ10.

I have observed a fairly consistent pattern of improvement in my patients. However, most do not have the miraculous improvement that my wife had. The most common comment I get at the two-month, follow-up exam is that their thinking and ability to concentrate have significantly improved. They feel that they have come out of their mental fog. At the four-month exam, they state that they are usually sleeping better and noticing some improvement in their energy level. The last things to improve are the pain, fever, and frequent infections.

BIONUTRITION

Their immune system is definitely improved, which is evidenced by the decrease in the number infections they have and the frequency of swollen glands and fevers that they suffer. The medical literature shows us that we can improve our immune systems via nutritional supplements, as explained in Chapter 9. Keep in mind, however, this usually takes a minimum of six months.

My patients do suffer setbacks, and not all of them show improvement. Increased stress levels, infections, surgeries, or injuries always seem to delay or prohibit any improvement. Some patients just do not improve, but 60 to 70 percent of my patients are having good to excellent results. That is better than the 0 percent improvement that I was having prior to using nutritional supplementation. They are returning to a functional life style, even though they are still not totally over their illness. If I am able to start working with a patient earlier in the course of their illness, I have better results. Patients who are willing to improve their diet and willing to exercise carefully also seem to do better.

I have treated more than 80 patients with fibromyalgia/chronic fatigue syndrome in my office and have been involved clinically with over 400 other patients across the country. They are all experiencing the same results. The results have been encouraging, and many of these patients are now functioning at a much better level. They still need to be careful, since they are definitely vulnerable to any stressful situation in their lives. However, if they have a setback, they have learned to increase their antioxidant intake for a week or two and be a little more careful with their schedule.

A REAL-LIFE STORY

One of my patients shared this story with me:

My personal experience with fibromyalgia began in November of 1990. I had been a person who seldom became sick, but that year I became very ill with flu-like symptoms that caused my body to ache to the point where I thought I would have to be rushed to the emergency room at the local hospital. My body ran a fever for two days, fluctuating between 101 and 102 degrees. It took almost two weeks before I recovered fully from this virus.

I spent one spring day in 1991 outdoors doing yard work – not an unusual task for me. But when I awoke the next morning, I felt as if I had moved furniture for three days. My thought was that I had probably just overdone it the day before. Little did I realize that this was only the beginning of uncomfortable feelings.

The next problem I encountered was sleep disorder. Although I tried a number of solutions, such as Tylenol PM, less coffee, and warm milk, nothing seemed to help. I continued to struggle with erratic sleep patterns for the next four years. I also experienced confusion, memory loss, and visual disturbances during this period of time. It wasn't long after that I became aware of the joint pain, knots in my shoulders, headaches, and a sore throat. The joint pain and the knots in my shoulders were more apparent in the morning hours; the sore throat and mild headaches were a constant problem. I realized that something very serious was affecting the quality of my health.

When I began waking each morning with stiffness, I knew it was time to seek medical help. At this point, I was getting only three to four hours of sleep night, and those few hours were not restful. It seemed as if my nerves were frayed, and every little noise and action irritated them.

The medication Dr. Strand gave me enabled my sleeping pattern to change somewhat, but after using the medication for a year, I started to develop side effects. This particular medication caused my heart to race and gave me extreme mood swings and horrid nightmares. I was convinced that the medication was doing more harm than good, so I decided to stop taking it.

It was time for a checkup with Dr. Strand, and I was feeling uncomfortable about telling him that I threw away his medicine and was trying vitamin therapy. He always told me if we ate properly, we could get all the nutrients we needed from our food. To my surprise, he had recently become involved in studies concerning the effects of antioxidants in the healing process. He placed me on an aggressive nutritional-supplement program.

In September of 1995, I started this program of nutritional supplements. The effects were amazing! Within three weeks I noticed a significant energy surge. No longer did I have to go to bed at 8:30 in order to make it through another day. Shortly after feeling more energy, I became aware that the painful knots in my shoulder blades had disappeared. By November, the joint and muscle aches started to subside.

In December I had some minor surgery. Some of the symptoms returned shortly afterward. I increased my antioxidant intake, and within two weeks the symptoms were no longer a problem. In March of 1996, I slept my first eight hours. And I noticed that my sleep pattern was once again the normal deep sleep I had previously enjoyed. My nerves were no longer frayed, and I felt a pervasive sense of wellness returning. Confusion cleared and my thinking process began to improve.

It has been two years now, and I am still doing well.

SECTION II

Thirteen

Bionutrition versus Recommended Dietary Allowances

The recommended dietary allowances were developed originally starting in the 1920s and 1930s simply as a minimal requirement on intake of 10 essential nutrients in order to avoid acute deficiency diseases. Acute deficiency diseases are like rickets (deficiency in vitamin D), pellagra (deficiency in niacin), and scurvy (deficiency in vitamin C). Therefore, if you took in at least the recommended dietary allowance of these essential nutrients, you would avoid developing one of these acute deficiency diseases. RDAs were also used as a baseline nutritional requirement for normal growth and development. RDAs have done their job. In 26 years of clinical practice, I have never seen any of these acute deficiency diseases. In fact, the Center for Disease Control does not even track these diseases anymore, since they are so rarely seen.

The United States government now requires all food and supplement labeling to use the RDAs as their standard. This has elevated the RDAs in the minds of almost all physicians and lay people alike. However, after you begin to become

However, after you begin to become familiar with the medical literature in regards to nutritional supplementation and its effect on chronic degenerative disease, you become convinced of one overriding truth – RDAs have absolutely nothing to do with chronic degenerative diseases.

familiar with the medical literature in regards to nutritional supplementation and its effect on chronic degenerative disease, you become convinced of one overriding truth – RDAs have absolutely nothing to do with chronic degenerative diseases. I believe this one simple truth is the cause of more confusion about the health benefits of nutritional supplementation than absolutely any other truth. Physicians are trained to believe that the RDAs are the level of nutrients needed to prevent acute deficiency diseases as well as the level of nutrients needed by the body to maintain health in general. This false assumption by physicians, registered dieticians, and nutritionists alike is the reason I believe nutritional supplementation is receiving such resistance by the medical profession. There are other reasons, but I believe this is a major reason.

RDAs, as I stated earlier, have absolutely nothing to do with chronic degenerative diseases. Studies that are appearing in our medical literature are establishing totally different levels of nutrients that are needed to help prevent or at least reduce the risk of these chronic degenerative diseases. These are the studies that physicians keep demanding are necessary for them to consider changing their minds. Well, the studies are here. Many of them are well referenced in this book. But we as physicians and health care providers choose to ignore them and misinterpret their importance for our patients. Bionutrition is taking these nutrients at the optimal levels that have been shown to provide a health benefit in the medical literature. Therefore, bionutrition has nothing to do with RDAs.

The best example that I feel illustrates this point is vitamin E. The RDA of vitamin E is 10 to 15 IU, depending on the sex and age of the patient. The medical literature does not even begin to show a health benefit from vitamin E supplementation until you start using at least 100 IU. This health benefit increases all the way up to 400 IU. Future studies may demonstrate improved health benefits with even greater amounts of vitamin E supplementation. However, for now most physicians who are familiar with the medical literature regarding vitamin E supplementation are now recommending that their patients take 400 IU of vitamin E in supplementation. This is because 400 IU of vitamin E is now felt to be the optimal level of intake for this nutrient. This is certainly significantly different from the RDA level of vitamin E, which is 10 to 15 IU.

SO WHY DON'T WE JUST EAT THE RIGHT FOODS?

For 23 years I told my patients that if they would just go out and eat the right foods, they did not need nutritional supplements. I made this statement based on the presumption (which I believed) that all you needed was the RDA level of all these nutrients. Obviously, the medical literature has changed my mind, but what about all the other physicians that you hear make this statement? Well, I agree with them about the fact that you do need to eat the right foods. By merely eating five to seven servings of fruits and vegetables a day, you lower your risk of nearly every cancer two to threefold. If you include a low-fat, high-fiber diet with your fruits and vegetables, you also significantly reduce your risk of heart attack, stroke, cancer, diabetes, and a host of other chronic degenerative diseases. This is not a bad place to start. I always explain to my patients that they must supplement a good diet, not a bad one.

Unfortunately, most Americans do not eat this way. We take in about 38 to 40 percent of calories in fat, most of which is saturated. We spend more money at fast food restaurants than we do at grocery stores. The medical journal Pediatrics, in its September 1997 issue, reported that only one percent of the children in the United States get the proper recommended nutrients from their diet (this is using RDA levels).[2] Poor eating habits in childhood usually persist into poor eating habits as adults. The Second National Health and Nutritional Survey (NHANES II) examined about 12,000 American adults and evaluated their eating habits.[3]

Here are some of their findings:

1. Seventeen percent of the population did not eat any vegetables.
2. If you excluded potatoes and salads, 50 percent of the population did not eat any vegetables. In other words, only half of the population ate "garden" vegetables.
3. Only 41 percent had any fruit or fruit juices.
4. Only nine percent of the population met the USDA guidelines of eating a minimum of five servings of fruits and vegetables a day. Among Blacks, there were only five percent that ate the recommended amount of fruits and vegetables.

There is also another major problem today, and that involves concern about the quality of the food we are eating. Because of the way we produce and preserve our food today, this is a very real concern. Rex Beach wrote in his report to the U.S. Senate:

"Do you know that most of us today are suffering from certain dangerous diet deficiencies which cannot be remedied until the depleted soils from which our foods come are brought into proper mineral balance? The alarming fact is that foods – fruits and vegetables and grains – now being raised on millions of acres of land that no longer contain enough of certain minerals are starving us, no matter how much we eat." [5]

The interesting thing about this quote was that it was given to the Seventy-fourth Congress in 1936. Since that time, we have done nothing to improve the situation; in fact, the situation is much worse. Our fertilizers are only putting back potassium, nitrogen, and phosphorous. There are five major minerals (calcium, magnesium, chloride, phosphorous, and potassium) and at least 16 trace minerals that are essential for optimal health. Plants cannot create minerals. They must absorb them from the soil. If our soils do not have the minerals, our plants will not have them either. Farmers are more concerned about bushels per acre than the nutrient content of the food they produce. Economics is the driving force.[5]

There is little argument today that the quality of our foods have declined when compared to our foods of other generations. Our food industry has been able to make available a wide variety of fruits and vegetables throughout the year. The variety is good. However, they are available at a sacrifice. Green harvesting means picking fruits and vegetables before they are mature. Making foods available all year round and shipping food over long distances requires cold storage and other preservation methods, which allow for the depletion of vital nutrients. Our food is also highly processed. The refinement process of our flour to create white bread removes more than 23 essential nutrients, magnesium being one of the most important. Our food industry then puts back about eight of these nutrients into our bread and calls it "enriched." Convenience and ease of preparation offered by our highly processed food is definitely offset by the lack of nutritional value and the preservatives needed to extend their shelf life.

It is a fact that our foods are significantly depleted of vital nutrients, even at the time we purchase them; however, more nutrients are lost in the preparation of our foods. Overcooking, delay in preparing fresh foods, and freezing our foods are some of the reasons our foods lose nutritional value when we prepare them. For example:

1. Fresh salads and cut vegetables and fruits lose more than 40 to 50 percent of their value if they sit for more than three hours.

2. More than 80 percent of the magnesium is lost when we remove the germ (outer portion of the grain) in the process of making white flour.

3. Vitamin C is vulnerable to both heat and cold and is significantly depleted with prolonged storage.

4. Folic acid is significantly lost during the preparation of food.

These are all good arguments for people to consider when trying to decide whether they need to be taking nutritional supplements or not. However, when you try to provide the body with optimal levels of these nutrients, it becomes readily apparent that supplementation is the only option. For example, in order to get the 400 IU of vitamin E each day (which we believe is the optimal level), you would have to eat 33 pounds of spinach, or 27 pounds of butter, or 5 pounds of wheat germ, or 2 1/2 pounds of almonds. Does this sound a little impractical?

I have several patients who have become very proactive after losing their health. They buy everything that is organically grown. They eat a great diet and they exercise. However, there is absolutely no way that they can achieve the benefits that patients achieve when they take nutritional supplements at these optimal levels. They are doing the right thing, but they still need to supplement their great diet.

In order to get the level of antioxidants, minerals, and vitamin B cofactors required to protect us against oxidative stress, these nutrients must be supplemented. Remember: bionutrition is providing the body with the optimal level of these micronutrients. These are not RDA levels but the level of nutrients that have been shown in current medical literature to provide the best protection against long-term, chronic degenerative diseases.

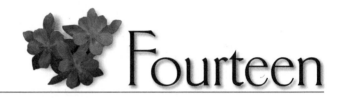

Fourteen

Nutritional Supplements

In the first part of the book, we looked at oxidative stress and how it affects the body. By looking at individual diseases, we are able to gain an understanding of the rationale behind using nutritional supplements. In this second part of the book, we are going to look at each individual nutrient and see how it plays a role in the overall recommendations for a supplementation program. Therefore, we will first detail each vitamin and nutrient to gain a better understanding of their particular role in the body. Then, I will put it all together so that you can understand the principles of nutritional supplementation.

Vitamins are essential for the body and are nutrients the body just can't make. We need to get our vitamins and minerals from our food. As I explained earlier, our foods are depleted of these essential nutrients, and the levels we need to fight oxidative stress are much greater than we could ever get from our food.

There are 13 different vitamins that are broken down into fat-soluble (vitamins A, D, E, and K) and water-soluble vitamins (vitamin C and the B vitamins). There are several other important antioxidants we need in both our diet and supplement program to maximize our fight against free radicals. In the next chapter, we will discuss in detail the minerals that are essential to any supplement program.

FAT-SOLUBLE VITAMINS
VITAMIN A (RETINOL) AND THE CAROTENOIDS

Vitamin A is a fat-soluble vitamin that is important in the function of the eye, mucous membranes, immune system, and skin. It helps to make the visual purple of your eye, which is necessary for night vision. The best food sources of vitamin A are liver, kidney, butter, milk, and fish oils. The RDA of vitamin A is 5,000 IU, or as measured by its new method, 1,000 retinol equivalents. However, there is concern with supplementation of vitamin A because of its toxic effect on the liver.[1] It has also been shown to cause birth defects when taken in excess in women who are pregnant.[2] Therefore, I tend to stay away from straight vitamin A as a supplement. If you do take vitamin A, women in their child bearing years should take no more than 2,500 IU (800 retinol equivalents), and men should not take more than 5,000 IU (1,500 retinol equivalents) per day.

BETA-CAROTENE AND MIXED CAROTENOIDS

Carotenes are the most widespread pigments in nature. They are intensely colored and are also fat soluble. They create the tremendous colors seen in our fruits and vegetables. Their uniqueness lies in the fact that they are very safe to take in supplementation and become vitamin A in the body as the body has need for vitamin A. They also offer tremendous antioxidant activity. Therefore, there is no toxic buildup of vitamin A, and you have added antioxidant protection. There are more than 600 different carotenoids that can be found in our food supply. Beta-carotene is the most widely studied and most widely used carotenoid in nutritional supplements. There are high concentrations found in green, leafy vegetables and also in orange-colored fruits and vegetables.

In general, the carotenoids exert a much greater antioxidant activity than vitamin A.[3] Supplements that offer mixed carotenoids have a much better protective effect against free radicals than those using beta-carotene alone. The supplement should have 15,000 to 25,000 IU of beta-carotene.

The benefits of supplementation with carotenoids include the following:
1. Beta-carotene enhances our immune system.[4]
2. All carotenoids function as potent antioxidants, able to incorporate themselves into the cell membrane like vitamin E.[5]

3. Beta-carotene has been shown in several epidemiological studies to lower the risk of several different cancers (lung, cervix, skin, uterus, oral, and gastrointestinal tract).[6]
4. High levels of beta-carotene have been shown to significantly decrease your risk of heart attack (close to 40 percent).[7]
5. High levels of beta-carotene decrease the risk of developing age-related macular degeneration and cataracts.[8]
6. Lutein and zeaxanthin are carotenoids that accumulate in the retina of the eye, and their pigment protects the retina and macula from oxidative stress. This decreases the risk of macular degeneration.[9]
7. Beta-carotene and several of the carotenoids become vitamin A as the body needs them. Therefore, they are a safe way to get all the vitamin A that you need.
8. Mixed carotenoids increase the resistance of LDL cholesterol to becoming oxidized.[10]

VITAMIN D (CHOLECALCIFEROL)

Our bodies are able to make vitamin D by the action of the sunlight on our skin. Vitamin D is essential for our bone health because it is absolutely necessary for the absorption of calcium. There are actually three different kinds of vitamin D, all of which exert various levels of activity on calcium metabolism. Vitamin D3 (cholecalciferol) is converted first in the liver and then the kidney into the most potent form of vitamin D. Good natural sources of vitamin D are cod liver oil, fish, butter, and egg yolks. As we grow older and are not in the sunlight as much, it is easy to develop vitamin D deficiency. The RDA of vitamin D is 200 IU. You should supplement with vitamin D3 (cholecalciferol) at a level of 500 to 800 IU daily. This is a safe level of supplementation.

Vitamin D is not only essential for our bone health but also has been shown to decrease our risk of both colon cancer and breast cancer.[11]

VITAMIN E (ALPHA-TOCOPHEROL)

Vitamin E is a fat-soluble vitamin and probably the most important antioxidant found in the body. Because it is fat soluble, it is the most important antioxidant within the cell membrane. This unique characteristic is what gives vitamin E its great protection to LDL cholesterol against oxidation. Along with the carotenoids, it is actually incorporated right into the cell membrane of LDL cholesterol. Wherever the LDL goes, the vitamin E goes along with it. It is crucial in the antioxidant defense system. The RDA of vitamin E is 10 to 15 IU. The most common food sources of vitamin E are seeds, nuts, whole grains, and vegetable oils. To provide the maximum level of protection against oxidative stress, we need to supplement our diet with at least 400 IU of vitamin E. The best form of vitamin E supplementation is the natural form, d-alpha-tocopherol. It's easy to confuse this with the synthetic form, which is dl-alpha-tocopherol. The synthetic form may actually inhibit the natural form from entering the cell membrane. Therefore, I recommend supplementing only with the natural form. Use d-alpha-tocopherol succinate for the best results.

The benefits of vitamin E supplementation include the following:

1. Vitamin E offers great protection against heart attack and stroke because it significantly increases the resistance of LDL cholesterol to oxidative modification.[12]
2. Vitamin E lowers insulin resistance and improves diabetic control.[13]
3. Low levels of vitamin E have been shown to increase the risk of getting certain kinds of cancer, especially cancers of the gastrointestinal tract.[14]
4. Vitamin E prevents platelet aggregation. This is the same mechanism that gives aspirin its effectiveness against heart disease. When vitamin E and aspirin are taken together, this effect is actually enhanced and is believed to reduce heart attacks even more.[15]
5. Vitamin E boosts the immune system, especially in the elderly.[16]
6. Vitamin E's antioxidant activity makes it one of the most important nutrients in the war against degenerative disease.

VITAMIN K (PHYLLOQUINONE)

Vitamin K is a fat-soluble vitamin essential in the manufacturing of clotting factors. Coumadin (warfarin) is the blood-thinning drug taken by many people. It works by inhibiting vitamin K's ability to make blood-clotting factors, and it prolongs the prothrombin time. As mentioned in the chapter on osteoporosis, vitamin K is very important in the development of new bone. It is essential in the conversion of osteocalcin to its active form. This allows calcium to be deposited in the bone. It is, therefore, a critical nutrient in the prevention of osteoporosis.

Some of the best food sources of vitamin K are dark leafy green vegetables, broccoli, lettuce, cabbage, and spinach. The RDA for vitamin K varies, depending on your weight, but it ranges from 50 to 80 mcg per day. Vitamin K should be taken in supplementation in the range of 50 to 100 mcg per day. I have patients who are on Coumadin taking vitamin K supplementation. As long as they take their supplements on a consistent basis and their vitamin K supplement is in this recommended dose, there is no problem maintaining their protime at a therapeutic level. Most physicians prefer that their patients not take vitamin K with Coumadin. Therefore, you should consult your physician about taking vitamin K if you are also taking Coumadin.

WATER-SOLUBLE VITAMINS
VITAMIN C (ASCORBIC ACID)

Vitamin C is a water-soluble vitamin. This makes it an ideal antioxidant that primarily works within the water environments of the body, which may be both inside and outside the cell. As a vitamin its major role is the manufacturing of collagen, which is an essential protein substance of the body.

The best food sources of vitamin C are citrus fruits, but vitamin C is also found in broccoli, potatoes, and Brussels sprouts. The present RDA for vitamin C is 60 mg per day. However, there has been a significant amount of discussion about raising this to 200 mg per day. Vitamin C supplementation has been the most common vitamin supplement in America. This is due in a large part to the research of Linus Pauling.

The documented benefits of vitamin C are primarily because of its potent antioxidant activity and ability to boost the immune system. Medical literature shows us that in order to get the best results from supplementation of vitamin C, we need to supplement with more – between one to two grams of vitamin C each day. There is good evidence that patients with chronic degenerative diseases should consider taking even more than two grams a day. Ascorbic acid is the most common form of vitamin C supplementation. However, the calcium, zinc, magnesium, and potassium ascorbates are absorbed better and have increased antioxidant activity. Ester-C has been promoted as the most effective vitamin C; however, I do not believe that the medical research supports this claim. Its cost is much higher also.

The benefits of vitamin C supplementation are as follows:

1. Vitamin C has been shown to improve lung function in asthma, emphysema, and cystic fibrosis.[17]
2. It is the most potent antioxidant protecting the oxidation of LDL cholesterol within the plasma. It also regenerates vitamin E. Many studies have shown that individuals with the highest vitamin C levels have the lowest incidence of coronary artery disease.[18]

BIONUTRITION

3. Vitamin C elevates HDL cholesterol.[19]
4. It lowers blood pressure.[19]
5. There is a significant decrease in the risk of several cancers, especially lung, gastrointestinal, cervical, and pancreatic cancers.[20]
6. It decreases the incidence of cataracts and macular degeneration.[21,22]
7. It enhances the immune system.[23]

VITAMIN B1 (THIAMIN)

Vitamin B1 is a water-soluble vitamin that is essential in the utilization of carbohydrates. This vitamin is needed for the body to maintain energy. There is very little storage of this nutrient, so it needs to be provided every day. Rich plant sources of thiamin are soybeans, brown rice, sunflower seeds, and peanuts. Other good sources of thiamin include breads and nuts.

The RDA of vitamin B1 is 1.5 mg per day. Vitamin B1 should be supplemented at 20 to 30 mg daily.

Thiamin, along with other B vitamins, is important in the supportive role of antioxidant activity. It is also very important in memory and our ability to think. There are studies which show that it mimics the effect of acetylcholine in the brain.[24] This may explain why studies that have used vitamin B1 in supplementation have shown clinical improvement in patients with Alzheimer's dementia.[25] Mental function has improved in other situations, but it has been best documented in patients with the chronic use of dilantin in seizures.

VITAMIN B2 (RIBOFLAVIN)

Vitamin B2 is important in the production of energy as well as in the regeneration of glutathione, one of the key intracellular antioxidants. Food sources of vitamin B2 are mushrooms, organ meats, almonds, wild rice, and green leafy vegetables.

The RDA of vitamin B2 is 1.7 mg daily. Your supplement should contain at least 25 to 35 mg daily.

Riboflavin is essential because of its support of the antioxidant system, especially glutathione. The synergistic effect of these nutrients on optimal antioxidant function cannot be overemphasized.

VITAMIN B3 (NIACIN)

Niacin is important as a cofactor for many enzymatic functions in the body. It is important in the production of energy and in fat and cholesterol metabolism.

The best food sources for niacin are meats, fish, legumes, whole grains, and milk.

The RDA of niacin is 20 mg daily. Supplementation should be 40 to 50 mg daily. There is a pharmacological effect when niacin is used in very high doses. Safety of this approach is discussed in a later chapter. In well-controlled studies, niacin in the range of 1.5 to 4.5 grams daily showed a 23 percent reduction in LDL cholesterol (bad cholesterol) and a 33 percent increase in HDL cholesterol (good cholesterol).[26] The niacin was increased slowly over a four-month period of time. I am impressed with the elevation of HDL cholesterol. This is very difficult to increase in clinical medicine. Niacin has its drawbacks in liver toxicity and the skin flushing it causes.

VITAMIN B5 (PANTOTHENIC ACID)

Vitamin B5 is important in the production of energy, hormones, and neurotransmitters. Deficiencies in vitamin B5 are rare. Good sources of vitamin B5 include milk, fish, poultry, whole grains, sweet potatoes, and oranges.

The RDA of vitamin B5 is 5 to 7 mg daily. Supplementing with 90 to 120 mg daily is important for energy production and glucose handling, especially in diabetics.

VITAMIN B6 (PYRIDOXINE)

Vitamin B6 is an important, water-soluble vitamin involved in the formation of many of the body's proteins and neurotransmitters of the nervous system. It also is needed in the formation of hemoglobin for red blood cells and for maintaining proper hormonal balance and immune function.

Food sources include whole grains, bananas, nuts, potatoes, and cauliflower. The RDA of vitamin B6 is 2 mg daily. Supplementation should be with 20 to 30 mg of pyridoxine hydrochloride each day. Vitamin B6 levels are linked to having adequate levels of magnesium.

Vitamin B6 is needed in the proper functioning of over 60 enzyme systems, many of which are involved in our antioxidant defense systems. Also, vitamin B6 is involved in the production of all the neurotransmitters in the brain.

The benefits of vitamin B6 supplementation are as follows:

1. There has been significant improvement in asthma patients who take B6 supplements.[27]
2. There has been significant decrease in the risk of heart disease, primarily because B6 helps decrease the levels of homocysteine.[28]

BIONUTRITION

3. There has been significant improvement in the pain of patients with carpal tunnel syndrome.[29]
4. Vitamin B6 has been shown to be very low in depressed patients, especially women who are taking birth control pills or estrogen. These individuals improve with vitamin B6 supplementation.[30]
5. There is improvement and protection against peripheral nerve pain in diabetics.[31]
6. Vitamin B6 prevents recurrent kidney stones in patients with a high risk of developing calcium oxalate kidney stones.[32]
7. It decreases the risk of osteoporosis because of improved homocysteine metabolism. (See Chapter 11)
8. It improves premenstrual syndrome symptoms.[33]

VITAMIN B12 (COBALAMIN)

Vitamin B12 is an important B vitamin that acts with folic acid in many enzyme systems involved in the formation of DNA, red blood cells, and the myelin sheath around nerves. In order for the body to absorb B12, the body needs to secrete a special digestive enzyme in the stomach called intrinsic factor.

Vitamin B12 is found in significant amounts only in animal products, such as eggs, meat, fish, and cheese. The RDA for vitamin B12 is 2 mcg per day. Supplementation should be 50 to 75 mcg daily.

The benefits of vitamin B12 supplementation include the following:
1. Vitamin B12 decreases the risk of vascular disease because of its importance in homocysteine metabolism.[34]
2. It has been shown to improve impaired mental function in the elderly.[35]
3. It improves the symptoms of depression.[36]

FOLIC ACID

Folic acid is an important B vitamin that is essential for DNA synthesis. Without adequate levels of folic acid, cells just do not divide properly.

Foods high in folic acid include green leafy vegetables, legumes, broccoli, cabbage, whole grains, and oranges. The RDA of folic acid is 200 mcg daily; supplementation with folic acid should be 1,000 mcg daily. This level is essential to provide the body with the optimal levels of folic acid needed for protection against cancer and vascular disease.

The benefits of folic acid supplementation include the following:

1. Folic acid decreases the risk of heart attack and stroke because of its ability to lower homocysteine levels.[37]
2. It helps prevent neural tube defects in newborns.[38]
3. It decreases the risk of osteoporosis because of improvement in homocysteine metabolism.[39]
4. It decreases the risk of cancer.[40]
5. It improves depression and mental confusion, especially in the elderly.[41]

CHOLINE

Choline is essential in the manufacture of acetylcholine, an important neurotransmitter, and for the metabolism of fat. Choline can be manufactured from methionine metabolism but has been designated an essential nutrient.

Choline is found in legumes, whole grains, lettuce, and cauliflower. No RDA has been established for choline. Supplementation should be 100 to 125 mg daily. Choline supplementation has been shown to increase acetylcholine levels in the brain. This is very important in Alzheimer's dementia.[42]

INOSITOL

Inositol is similar to choline, and supplementation has been beneficial even though the body is able to make it. It promotes the export of fat from the liver. It is a primary component of cell membranes. It is important for the proper function of nerve, brain, and muscle.

Inositol is present mainly as a fiber component known as phytic acid. Good plant sources of inositol are whole grains, citrus fruits, nuts, and legumes.

Inositol is necessary for the proper function of several neurotransmitters. This is just one of the important nutrients needed in a supplementation program. Inositol should be supplemented at 100 to 200 mg daily.

COENZYME Q10 (UBIQUINONE)

CoQ10 is a vitamin-like substance that also has potent antioxidant activity. It is essential for the production of energy within the mitochondria (battery of the cell). Studies show that it is probably the most important nutrient necessary for the production of ATP, which is the source of energy for the body.[43]

CoQ10 is found in almost every food, although this is not sufficient to produce the clinical effects that high doses of CoQ10 supplementation can achieve. Supplementation of CoQ10 should be in the range of 15 to 30 mg in healthy

BIONUTRITION

individuals. Higher levels of CoQ10 have been discussed earlier for particular medical situations.

The benefits of CoQ10 supplementation are as follows:

1. CoQ10 improves heart function in cardiomyopathy and congestive heart failure. [44]
2. It enhances the immune system.[45]
3. It causes inhibition and regression of breast cancer.[46]
4. It improves mitral valve prolapse.[47]
5. It improves angina.[48]
6. It increases the muscular strength of patients with muscular dystrophy.[49]

BIOTIN

Biotin is a B vitamin essential in the manufacture of fats and glycogen and is important in energy production because of its improved utilization of sugar.

Important food sources include eggs, nuts, cheese, and soybeans. It is manufactured in the intestines by gut bacteria.

The RDA of biotin is 30 mcg daily. Supplementation should be between 50 to 100 mcg daily.

Biotin supplementation has been shown to improve insulin sensitivity.[50] Higher doses in diabetics have been shown not only to decrease insulin needs but also to improve damaged nerves.[51]

GLUTATHIONE AND N-ACETYL L-CYSTEINE

The body makes glutathione from N-acetyl L-cysteine. The glutathione antioxidant system is the most important antioxidant system within the cell. It has been shown that the levels of glutathione may be increased by supplementation with N-acetyl L-cysteine.[52] Therefore, a good supplementation program should include the important nutrients that are required to synthesize glutathione within the body. These are niacin, vitamin B2, and selenium.

The benefit of increasing the intracellular antioxidant glutathione is that oxidative stress may be better brought back into balance. This is important in preventing or at least decreasing the incidence of chronic degenerative diseases.

BIOFLAVONOID ANTIOXIDANTS

Now that we understand the basis of chronic degenerative disease, there is an ongoing search for antioxidants that will give us an even better advantage when trying to bring this oxidative stress back into balance. There will be intense research to try to find the most potent antioxidants and combinations of antioxidants. There are several thousand bioflavonoid antioxidants that can be found in our food. Their antioxidant activity may be accentuated by supplying these nutrients to the body in supplementation. Having seen the medical evidence – that antioxidants have great value in decreasing the risk of chronic degenerative diseases – it is understandable why nutritional supplement companies are trying to find the most potent antioxidants.

Quercetin, rutin, cruciferous, green tea extract, bilberry extract, and hesperidin are just a few of these antioxidants. Broccoli extract also contains sulforaphane, which is believed to have significant anticancer properties. By combining several of these bioflavonoid antioxidants, there are synergistic antioxidant and possibly cancer-inhibition effects.

The most potent antioxidants that I believe have been found to date are proanthocyanidins, also called pycnogenols. They come from either pine bark or grape seeds and are very potent. I personally prefer the grape-seed extract because I believe it is the more potent of the two.[53,54]

Supplementation of these bioflavonoids is best when taken in combination. Proanthocyanidins should be supplemented at about 100 mg daily. They are much more effective when combined with other antioxidants, especially vitamin C. In patients with chronic degenerative diseases, allergies, or fatigue syndromes, I usually recommend 100 to 400 mg daily. They are very safe and very effective at this level when used in addition to a complete, well-balanced, supplement program.

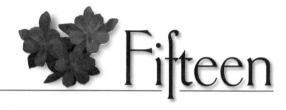

Fifteen

Mineral Supplementation

There are no more important nutrients to be supplemented than the minerals. Plants absorb minerals from the soil. As has been explained previously, however, there has been a tremendous depletion of minerals in our soil. Plants are not able to make minerals. If the soil does not have them, there is no way…the plants will be able to get them. I believe that the greatest nutritional deficiencies today are found in our minerals. If we do not have adequate levels of minerals available in our bodies, it doesn't matter how many antioxidants we have. The antioxidants will just be able to do their job, since they all need to have these minerals available for use in their enzymatic reactions.

CALCIUM

Calcium is the most abundant mineral in the body. The majority of calcium is in the bone. Calcium is also important in many enzyme systems in the body. It is important for the contraction of muscles, the release of our neurotransmitters, clotting ability, and for the regulation of the rhythm of the heart. Its importance in preventing and correcting osteoporosis was discussed in detail previously.

The primary food sources of calcium are dairy products. Plant foods that are good sources of calcium are spinach, kale, turnip greens, and other leafy green vegetables. The RDA of calcium is 1,200 mg per day. Supplementation of calcium is usually recommended to be from 800 to 1,500 mg per day. Most physicians agree with supplementing calcium since it is so hard to obtain these levels with diet alone.

When supplementing with calcium, you should understand which is the best form of calcium. Calcium citrate is the best supplement of calcium because it is the most easily absorbed and the most bioavailable. Calcium carbonate is the next best supplement; however, its absorption falls dramatically in patients who have low stomach acid. Unfortunately, the problem of low acid is very common in our elderly population, and these are the people who need calcium.[1] The FDA has cautioned people not to take calcium supplements that are derived from dolomite or bone meal because they may contain potentially high levels of lead.

Calcium levels have been found to be depleted in patients with hypertension. Studies have shown that some hypertension patients respond nicely to calcium supplements and some do not.[2]

MAGNESIUM

Magnesium is involved in more than 300 different enzyme systems in the body and is found primarily in the brain, heart, kidney, and liver. Magnesium deficiency is probably the most underdiagnosed deficiency in the body. Physicians check magnesium levels all the time, but we are only checking serum levels. Only 0.3 percent of the body's magnesium is found in the blood; the rest is found in the body's tissues. By the time low serum magnesium is noted, the body is severely depleted.

The best food sources of magnesium are tofu, seeds, nuts, whole grains, and green leafy vegetables. Flour refinement, which takes out all the magnesium, has led to a significant problem with magnesium deficiency. The RDA for magnesium is 350 mg per day. Supplementation should be at least 500 to 800 mg per day.

Magnesium is critical for many cellular functions, including energy production, cellular replication, and electrical conduction within the heart. More than 300,000 cardiac arrests a year have been attributed to magnesium deficiency.[3] When a patient is admitted to many of our coronary care units with a heart attack, he or she is given magnesium sulfate intravenously right away, since this has been shown to improve the survival of the patient.[4] In some studies, patients with cardiac arrhythmias improved over 50 percent of the time just on magnesium supplementation alone.[5]

Other benefits to magnesium supplementation include the following:
1. Magnesium supplementation improves asthma because the smooth muscles of the bronchial tree are able to relax.[6]
2. It improves survival with patients who suffer a heart attack.[4]
3. It improves high blood pressure.[7]
4. It improves mitral valve prolapse.[8]
5. It decreases the risk of diabetic retinopathy.[9]
6. It improves migraine and tension headaches.[10]
7. It improves osteoporosis.[11]
8. It improves the risk of preeclampsia in pregnancy.[12]
9. It helps alleviate premenstrual syndrome symptoms.[13]

ZINC

Zinc is an important mineral essential in the function of many hormones (insulin, growth hormone, and sex hormones). It is involved in more than 200 different enzymatic reactions.

The best-known food source of zinc is oysters, but it is also found in other shellfish, meats, and fish. There are good amounts in plant food such as grains, legumes, and nuts. The RDA of zinc is 15 mg daily. Supplementation should be with 20 to 30 mg of a chelated mineral or a zinc picolinate.

Zinc is heavily involved in our immune system. Studies have showed a modest supplementation of 20 mg of zinc in a group of elderly patients produces a significant increase in immune function.[14] Zinc supplementation may also increase a low sperm count.[15] Zinc has also shown protection against macular degeneration and improvement in Alzheimer's disease.[16,17]

BORON

Boron, as discussed in the chapter on osteoporosis, has been found to be necessary for the proper action of vitamin D. It also increases the endogenous (internal) excretion of the very active form of estrogen, 17 beta-estradiol.[18] This estrogen is great for bone preservation while very weak in its risk of cancer. It also has been found to give improvement to those individuals who have osteoarthritis.

BIONUTRITION

Fruits and vegetables are the main dietary source of boron. There is no RDA for boron. Supplementation should be 3 mg of boron daily, either in a chelated form or in a citrate or aspartate form.

CHROMIUM

Chromium is important for glucose metabolism. It significantly improves insulin sensitivity. This allows insulin to work more effectively and helps get glucose into the cell. Chromium has also been shown to help impaired glucose tolerance.[19]

Food sources of chromium include grains and meats. There is no RDA for chromium. Supplementation should be 200 to 300 mcg daily. Chromium picolinate is the best form to take.

IODINE

Iodine is required in the manufacture of thyroid hormone. There are few deficiencies today, thanks to iodized salt. The RDA is 150 mcg per day. Supplementation should be 100 to 200 mcg daily.

COPPER

Copper is an essential trace mineral necessary for several enzyme systems. It is needed for proper absorption of iron and for the proper formation of collagen. Its greatest importance, however, is in the proper functioning of the superoxide dismutase (SOD) antioxidant system.

The best food sources include shellfish, legumes, and split peas. The RDA for copper is 3 mg per day. Supplementation of this trace mineral is important. A chelated copper is best and should be somewhere between 3 to 6 mg daily.

SELENIUM

Selenium is a trace mineral needed in the enzymatic function of the glutathione peroxidase system. This antioxidant system is the most important antioxidant system within the cell.

There is significant selenium deficiency because this nutrient is so depleted in our soil. The RDA of selenium is 70 mcg per day. Supplementation is best with 200 mcg of a chelated form or the L-selenomethionine form.

There have been several documented benefits of selenium supplementation, including the following:

1. Selenium has been shown to decrease the risk of several types of cancer (prostate, colon, lung, and esophageal).[20]
2. It enhances several different aspects of the immune function.[21]
3. It decreases the risk of heart attack and stroke, especially where there had been a dietary deficiency.[22]
4. It improves the glutathione antioxidant system, which helps prevent or correct several chronic degenerative diseases but especially cataracts and rheumatoid arthritis.[23,24]

MANGANESE

Manganese is important in several enzyme reactions. It is involved in blood sugar control, energy metabolism, and in the antioxidant system superoxide dismutase (SOD).

Foods rich in manganese are nuts, whole grains, and green leafy vegetables.

The RDA of manganese is 5 mg daily. Supplementation should be 5 to 10 mg daily in a chelated form.

IRON

Iron is important in the formation of hemoglobin and in several enzyme systems involving energy production and DNA synthesis.

Our diets seem to have good sources of iron; hence, there is usually no problem with iron deficiency unless there is a source of blood loss. Once we absorb our iron, it is recycled and not eliminated from the body.

The RDA of iron is 12 to 15 mg per day. I recommend avoiding supplements with iron. Studies show an increased risk of heart attack in those individuals who have high iron intake.[25] These studies need to be confirmed. In the meantime, if you are going to take iron supplements, I advise taking no more than 10 to 15 mg of iron a day in supplementation.

MOLYBDENUM

This mineral is important in enzyme systems that detoxify sulfites and also in uric acid formation. Molybdenum in our food is directly related to its levels in our soil. It is important to supplement this mineral at 40 to 60 mcg daily. Molybdenum is important in detoxifying and in helping the body rid itself of cancer-causing chemicals.

BIONUTRITION

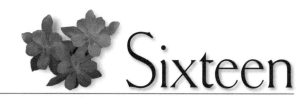

Sixteen

Safety of Nutritional Supplements

Throughout this book I related the medical evidence that demonstrates the effectiveness of nutritional supplements in preventing and/or slowing the progression of degenerative diseases. However, for these supplements to be effective for this purpose, they must be taken for a lifetime and they must be safe. Every time physicians prescribe a medication, especially if it is for the treatment of a chronic illness, we explain to the patient the potential danger in the use of that drug. It amazes me how many physicians try to get patients to quit taking their nutritional supplements because they feel that they could be danger-ous to their health. The medications we prescribe, according to Dr. Bruce Pomeranz, as reported in the April 15, 1998, Journal of the American Medical Association, cause over 100,000 deaths a year. He also states that another 2.1 million patients have serious complications because of properly prescribed medications. There have only been a handful of deaths reported in the last several decades because of supplements. These have been individuals who took many times the amount recommended in this book of a particular nutrient, such as niacin. Other situations involved accidental overdose of supplements, primarily in children. It is important to realize that nutritional supplements are not drugs but rather natural nutrients. Therefore, it is important to understand the safety of these nutrients at the optimal levels that are being recommended in this book.

When you understand the safety of these nutrients, you will begin to realize why vitamin and mineral supplements are ideal products to be used for chemoprevention and for reducing the risk of degenerative diseases. Pharmaceutical drugs may possess some clinical benefit in preventing some of these diseases, but they inherently create a risk to the patient. Nutritional supplements are simply nutrients that we get from our foods but at a higher level than is possible from food sources.

VITAMIN A

Of all the nutritional supplements, straight vitamin A causes the most concern. Vitamin A toxicity can occur in adults who take in excess of 50,000 IU per day for a prolonged period of time. (1) A lower dose may create toxicity if the patient has underlying liver disease. Signs of vitamin A toxicity include dry skin, brittle nails, hair loss, gingivitis, anorexia, nausea, fatigue, and irritability. Accidental ingestion of a single large dose of vitamin A by children (100,000 to 300,000 IU) can cause acute toxicity. This may present as headache, vomiting, and stupor because of the increase in intracranial pressure.[2]

Women must avoid vitamin A supplementation during pregnancy. Dosages as low as 5,000 to 10,000 IU are believed to have caused birth defects.[3]

I recommend to my patients that they not take straight vitamin A supplements because of these potential problems. The need for vitamin A within the body may be met by simply taking beta-carotene and the mixed carotenoids. These are very safe and the body is able to turn these into vitamin A as the need arises. Therefore, there is no toxic build up of vitamin A when you supplement with beta-carotene.

BETA-CAROTENE

Beta-carotene has been used in high doses over several years without a single reported adverse effect. Some individuals develop a yellowing of the skin called carotenodermia. However, this is totally benign and reverses completely once the beta-carotene is reduced or discontinued.

A recent study called the Alpha-Tocopherol Beta-Carotene Cancer Prevention Study conducted in Finland, and similar results repeated in Washington State, showed an actual, statistically significant, increased risk in the development of lung cancer in the group taking beta-carotene alone.[4] This was not observed in the patients who took vitamin E alone or in those who took this same level of beta-carotene along with vitamin E. This study involved males age 50 to 69 who had been heavy smokers for more than a 36-year period. This study has received great media coverage and has caught the attention of many physicians.

I loved to see these types of studies years ago so I could say to myself, "See, I was right all along. Vitamin supplements are dangerous to your health." Then I could ignore the next 20 studies that showed true health benefits from taking vitamins. If these studies are considered logically, one realizes that cancers develop over a 20-to-30-year period of time. The five to eight years these patients were followed was probably not long enough – especially given how much and how long the participants smoked.

These studies, however, should not be ignored. It is interesting to note those individuals who took both beta-carotene and vitamin E showed no increased risk. This raises the possibility that when beta-carotene is given in high doses alone, it actually may be a prooxidant (creates oxidative stress). When used in combination with vitamin E, this effect was not seen. Nevertheless, these studies stand in contrast to hundreds of clinical trials which have either shown a benefit or at least no harm. As I will explain in the next chapter, I do not believe in taking a particular supplement, like beta-carotene, in high doses alone.

VITAMIN E

Although vitamin E is a fat-soluble vitamin, it has a tremendous safety record. In clinical trials of vitamin supplementation, a dose as high as 3,200 IU per day has not shown any adverse effects. Vitamin E has been shown to inhibit platelet aggregation in much the same way as aspirin does.[5] This property of vitamin E is actually a benefit in reducing heart disease rather than a concern. Some researchers believe this will actually improve the effectiveness of aspirin in patients with heart disease.

VITAMIN C

Vitamin C is safe, even at very high doses, although some people may have abdominal bloating, gas, or diarrhea. At one point, there was a concern that vitamin C supplementation might increase the risk of kidney stones. This has been seen in only one clinical trial. There have now been four additional clinical trials that have not shown any increased risk of kidney stones in those patients who were taking vitamin C in supplementation.

VITAMIN D

Vitamin D has a great potential to cause toxicity. Dosages greater than 2000 IU are not recommended. In most cases, I do not recommend supplementing with vitamin D in doses greater than 500 to 800 IU per day. Vitamin D toxicity may increase the blood levels of calcium, causing deposits of calcium in internal organs and increasing the risk of kidney stones.[6]

NIACIN (VITAMIN B3)

Niacin supplementation may create flushing of the skin, nausea, and liver damage. Clinical studies have shown that slow-release products of niacin may decrease the risk of flushing, but they may also increase the risk of liver damage.[7]

Many people use high doses of niacin as a natural way to decrease their cholesterol levels. I recommend slowly building up to 1.5 grams per day. It is best to be under the direction of your physician.

VITAMIN B6 (PYRIDOXINE)

Vitamin B6 is one of the few water-soluble vitamins that carries a possible risk of toxicity. Doses greater than 2,000 mg can cause symptoms of nerve toxicity. When using doses between 50 to 100 mg daily, there have not been any reported cases of toxicity.[8]

FOLIC ACID

Folic acid supplementation may mask an underlying vitamin B12 deficiency. Therefore, you should always take vitamin B12 supplements when you are taking folic acid.

CHOLINE

Choline is generally well tolerated, although in very high doses (20 grams per day) it can create a fishy odor and cause some nausea, diarrhea, and abdominal pain.

CALCIUM

Calcium supplements are tolerated in doses up to 2,000 mg. It was once thought that high levels of calcium supplementation could lead to an increase in kidney stones; however, a recent study actually showed that higher levels of calcium intake actually decrease the risk of kidney stones. In other words, those individuals who had the lowest intake of calcium had the greatest risk of developing kidney stones.

IODINE

Iodine supplementation greater than 750 mcg can suppress thyroid hormone secretion. There have also been reports of acne-like skin eruptions at these higher levels of iodine intake.

IRON

There has been an increased concern about the use of iron in supplementation. The use of inorganic iron is even more of a concern. Americans generally get plenty of iron and supplementation of this nutrient may create an iron, overload, which has been associated with increased risk of heart disease in males. There is also some concern that iron may actually increase oxidative stress.

MANGANESE

Manganese taken in supplementation is very safe, although there are reports of people who develop manganese toxicity from their environment. This is usually seen in those who mine manganese or are exposed to high levels in the environment. These individuals may begin to hallucinate and become very irritable.

MOLYBDENUM

Molybdenum is quite safe. A daily intake of greater than 10 to 15 mg, however, may lead to gout-like symptoms.

SELENIUM

Selenium has been found to be safe in several clinical trials which used doses in the range of 400 to 500 mcg daily. I believe, however, that doses of selenium supplementation should be less than 300 mcg daily. Symptoms of selenium toxicity include depression, irritability, nausea, vomiting, and hair loss. (9)

There have been no toxic effects associated with supplementation of vitamin K, vitamin B1 (thiamin), vitamin B2 (riboflavin), biotin, vitamin B5 (pantethine), inositol, vitamin B12, chromium, silicon, CoQ10, boron, and alpha-lipoic acid.

Seventeen

Physician's Bias Against Nutritional Supplements

For the first 23 years of my clinical practice, I shared the popular physician view toward nutritional supplements. I told my patients that I felt nutritional supplements were a waste of their money and that they could obtain everything that they needed from their food. I believed that there weren't any significant medical studies that supported the use of nutritional supplements by my patients. So I can personally relate to the mind-set of probably well over 90 percent of the physicians in this country. Therefore, I believe that I am able to share with you where your physician is most likely coming from when it comes to nutritional supplementation, since I have been there.

Physicians are disease oriented and drug oriented. In medical school, we are primarily involved in learning about the diagnosis and treatment of disease states. Very little time is devoted to disease prevention, let alone nutrition. Most physicians believe that all their patients need are the RDA levels of these essential micronutrients, which they feel their patients can get from their diet.

This misconception was addressed in detail in Chapter 13. RDAs have become the standard by which physicians judge the nutritional supplementation industry. Most medical schools do not teach any nutrition to their medical students, and if they do teach any nutrition to their students, it is strictly on an elective basis. A recent survey of the medical schools showed that only 4% of the graduating physicians had any course in nutrition. This would usually be a course that would discuss the intake of proteins, fats, and carbohydrates. It would definitely not deal with nutritional supplementation. This is the main reason that I chose to call my book "Bionutrition." I wanted to emphasis the point that RDAs have absolutely nothing to do with chronic degenerative diseases. Bionutrition, on the other hand, is taking in these optimal levels of nutritional supplements that have been shown in our medical literature to provide a health benefit to our patients.

Nutritional supplementation is not about disease but about health. Patients are either trying to maintain their health or trying to gain back control of their health. Physicians have forgotten about the host (our bodies) when it comes to caring for patients. The results that I have seen since starting to recommend that my patients be taking high-quality nutritional supplements have been next to amazing. I am helping patients in ways that I was never able to before.

I have seen my share of quackery sold to my patients under the umbrella of alternative medicine. Before researching our medical literature, I always felt that nutritional supplements were used as an alternative to traditional medical care. I truly believed that nutritional supplements offered absolutely no health benefits to my patients and that they just cost my patients a lot of money. However, I now know that nutritional supplementation is NOT alternative medicine, but it is instead mainline traditional medicine. Most physicians just don't realize it. Nutritional supplementation is not about disease but about health. Patients are either trying to maintain their health or trying to gain back control of their health. Physicians have forgotten about the host (our bodies) when it comes to caring for patients. The results that I have seen since starting to recommend that my patients be taking high-quality nutritional supplements have been next to amazing. I am helping patients in ways that I was never able to before. The main principle I have learned is the fact that our bodies are the best defense against all of the chronic degenerative diseases – not my drugs. By simply building up my patients' natural antioxidant defense system and immune system with these optimal levels of nutrients, they are becoming healthier. The medical literature is demonstrating over and over that there are health benefits to patients who take nutritional supplements. However, physicians are just not applying these scientific principles to their everyday practices. Instead, most physicians are doing everything they can to discourage their patients from taking supplements. Physicians, after all, are the authority, and most patients do listen to our advice. It is sad when I think of all the patients who quit their supplements because of my advice. I was truly uniformed. However, that is not a good excuse.

When my colleagues begin to question why I recommend nutritional supplements to my patients, I respond by asking them a question: "Have you ever recommended to your patients that they begin an exercise program?" They usually respond by saying of course. Then I ask them, "WHY?" They state that they feel that their patients who have a regular exercise program have health benefits over those patients who do not. I ask them on what do they base that conclusion? They reply saying the medical literature. I then ask them are they treating a disease when they make this recommendation? They simply answer NO. I then ask if they have ever recommended that their patients eat a high-fiber, low-fat diet, making sure that they eat five to seven servings of fruits and vegetables each day? They almost all say, "Well, of course." I go through the same logic and usually get the same response. Again, I finish by asking them if they are treating a disease when they give this advice to their patients. They always say NO. Well, that is how I feel about nutritional supplements. I believe that my patients who take high-quality nutritional supplements have a health benefit over my patients who don't. The medical literature has convinced me of this truth. Just like I have been convinced by the medical literature that my patients who exercise and eat a healthy diet have a health benefit, I now believe that my patients who take nutritional supplements receive a tremendous health benefit. Am I treating a disease when I make this recommendation? ABSOLUTELY NOT. These are not drugs; they are simply nutrients that we should be getting from our food but at levels we cannot obtain from our food.

Many physicians do look at nutritional supplements as if they were drugs. I hear my colleagues say that they don't recommend supplements because they are not FDA approved. I respond by sharing with them that vitamin E, vitamin C, calcium, magnesium, and so forth are not drugs but natural nutrients that the body needs for everyday, normal, metabolic function. You simply are not able to get a patent from the FDA on natural nutrients. No drug company is going to spend millions of dollars trying to get a natural nutrient approved by the FDA. There is no money in it. They want to spend their money on getting their drugs approved by the FDA, because once that happens, it is like winning Lotto America. Remember: drugs actually change or block a natural metabolic function in order to produce a therapeutic effect. For example, calcium-channel blockers actually block the normal flow of calcium in and out of the cell, which causes the arteries to dilate and blood pressure to drop. Therefore, one of the therapeutic uses of calcium-channel blockers is with patients who have high blood pressure. These drugs, like all drugs, also have a long list of potential side effects, which are related to the changes they create in the body's normal metabolic function. Just spend some time looking at the Physician's Desk Reference (PDR), and it will become obvious that all drugs have potential risks as well as their therapeutic benefits. To the contrary, nutritional supplements are safe when taken at optimal levels.

Physicians truly do believe in nutritional supplementation – they just don't realize it. Since they look at these natural nutrients as drugs, and since they are disease oriented, that is the way they recommend them. For example, when a lady is entering menopause or has developed osteoporosis, the physician will recommend that she take calcium and vitamin D in supplementation. Many of my patients who have been diagnosed with coronary artery disease are advised by their cardiologist to start taking vitamin E and maybe vitamin C supplements. Physicians recommend that their women patients who are in their child bearing years should take folic acid supplements as a way to decrease their risk of having a baby with a neural tube defect, should they happen to get pregnant. Many of my patients leave the cardiologist's office on magnesium supplements when they are also being treated for rhythm problems with their heart. Some physicians are now even recommending to their patients who have cardiovascular disease that they should be taking folic acid, vitamin B12, and vitamin B6 in supplementation as an effective way to lower their homocysteine levels. These are just some of the examples where most physicians are in agreement that supplements are needed. They must not believe that they can get an adequate amount of these specific nutrients from their food, since they recommend that their patients take these supplements.

Physicians always tell me they want to see the double-blind clinical studies that show that patients need supplements. They truly believe that there is absolutely no scientific evidence for recommending supplements. I could have used thousands of scientific medical studies that have

This is the medical evidence that demands a verdict. Should you be taking nutritional supplements?

looked at the potential health benefits of supplements. I have referred to the major studies. Many of them are the well-controlled, double-blind, clinical trials that physicians demand to see. What better way to present my arguments to justify the recommendation of using nutritional supplements than with our own medical literature?

Physicians just need to become familiar with this medical literature that deals with nutritional supplements. This is the medical evidence that demands a verdict. Should you be taking nutritional supplements? Remember: nutritional supplementation is about health, not disease. The sooner physicians begin to realize this truth the sooner their patients will benefit. After all, physicians should be the authority on all health issues. Physicians owe it to themselves and their patients to be informed. This is our medical literature. Just because there will not be some pharmaceutical representative showing us these studies does not mean that we shouldn't take an objective look at them.

I have to admit that I was totally ignorant of these studies before I started my own research. Most physicians are uninformed about the health benefits that nutritional supplements can provide their patients. Someday the Surgeon General of the United States will issue a report on the health benefits that individuals may receive by taking nutritional supplements. It is just a matter of time. The findings in medical literature are simply just getting too strong to ignore any longer.

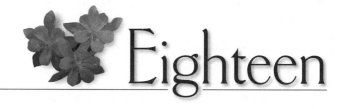

Eighteen

Bionutrition
PUTTING IT ALL TOGETHER

I am not a researcher or a nutritionist. I am a clinician. Therefore, when I look at the medical literature presented in this book, I look at it from a clinician's viewpoint. How can I best apply these principles to clinical medicine in order to help my patients? In other words, how do I apply this medical evidence to my everyday practice? The root cause of well over 50 chronic degenerative diseases has now been shown to be oxidative stress. This present generation is exposed to more emotional stress, pollutants, toxins, radiation, and drugs than any previous generation. This is the main reason we are seeing more chronic degenerative disease than we have ever seen before and at a much younger age. We simply have no choice but to live in this world and its environment. Accordingly, we must build up our antioxidant defense systems to their optimal levels. We simply must have enough antioxidants available to handle the number of free radicals our body produces. Today, because of nutritional science, we have the ability to provide these important antioxidants to the body at optimal levels because of the availability of quality nutritional supplements.

Bionutrition is the answer to "Winning the War Within." Bionutrition is simply defined as providing the essential antioxidant nutrients to the body at optimal levels that have been shown to provide a health benefit in the medical literature. It is simply a matter of balance. We need to have more antioxidants available than the number of free radicals our body produces. Nutritional supplementation is the answer.

Almost every study referred to in this book looked at just one nutrient and its effect on a particular disease. The most amazing fact to me was that the over-whelming majority of these studies showed a significant health benefit when using just one nutrient. There was an underlying principle that was very obvious to me throughout my research of the medical literature. These antioxidants work in synergy with one another. One plus one is not two, but eight or ten. Vitamin E is the best antioxidant within the cell membrane. Vitamin C is absolutely the best antioxidant within the plasma, and it regenerates vitamin E. Glutathione, along with its supporting nutrients selenium, riboflavin, niacin, and N-acetyl L-cysteine, work together to make up the most important antioxidant system functioning within the cell itself. Beta-carotene and the mixed carotenoids are very important free-radical scavengers. Alpha lipoic acid is both fat and water soluble and is able to work within both the plasma and the cell membrane. All of these antioxidants must have the antioxidant minerals selenium, copper, manganese, and magnesium available in adequate amounts in order to perform their job. Folic acid, vitamin B1, vitamin B2, vitamin B6, and vitamin B12 are also needed as cofactors in the enzymatic reactions of these antioxidants. What would happen if we gave our patients all of these nutrients together at these optimal levels? Once you begin to appreciate the devastating effect that oxidative stress has on our bodies, you begin to realize the fact that everyone needs all of these nutrients and at optimal levels.

What would happen if we gave our patients all of these nutrients together at these optimal levels? Once you begin to appreciate the devastating effect that oxidative stress has on our bodies, you begin to realize the fact that everyone needs all of these nutrients and at optimal levels.

As a clinician, I want my patients to have **ALL** the potential health benefits that nutritional supplements have been shown to offer. Therefore, I recommend that my patients take a complete, balanced, nutritional supplement that provides all of these nutrients at optimal levels. The cell is then able to decide what it

ANTIOXIDANTS	
Vitamin A	I prefer that all of my patients avoid taking straight vitamin A altogether. Supplementation of beta-carotene can be used instead of vitamin A.
Beta-carotene	15,000 to 25,000 IU daily
Vitamin C	1 to 2 grams daily as calcium, magnesium, zinc, or potassium ascorbates
Vitamin E	400 to 600 IU daily as d-alpha-tocopherol
Glutathione	10 to 20 mg daily
N-acetyl L-cysteine	60 to 75 mg daily
Alpha lipoic acid	15 to 20 mg daily
Coenzyme Q10	15 to 30 mg daily
Bioflavonoid complex	I recommend taking a combination of several bioflavonoids, which should include rutin, cruciferous, bilberry extract, green tea extract, broccoli concentrate, and quercetin; other combinations may also be effective. Mixed carotenoids zeaxanthin and lutein
Vitamin B complex	
Vitamin B1 (Thiamin)	20 to 30 mg daily
Vitamin B2 (Riboflavin)	25 to 35 mg daily
Vitamin B3 (Niacin)	40 to 50 mg daily
Vitamin B5 (Pantothenic acid)	90 to 120 mg daily
Vitamin B6 (Pyridoxine)	20 to 30 mg daily
Vitamin B12 (Cobalamin)	50 to 100 mcg daily
Folic acid	1,000 mcg daily
Choline	100 to 125 mg daily
Inositol	100 to 200 mg daily
Biotin	50 to 100 mcg daily
OTHER VITAMINS	
Vitamin D	500 to 800 IU daily as vitamin D3 (cholecalciferol)
Vitamin K	50 to 100 mcg daily
MINERALS	
Calcium	800 to 1,500 mg daily as calcium citrate
Magnesium	500 to 800 mg daily
Zinc	20 to 30 mg daily as zinc picolinate or chelated zinc
Boron	3 mg daily as chelated boron
Chromium	200 to 300 mcg daily as chromium picolinate

needs, and does not need. A proper nutritional supplement simply causes nutrients to work synergistically giving my patients the best opportunity to improve the body's chances for good health.

In addition to these nutrients, I also recommend that my patients take essential fatty acids (omega 3 and omega 6 fatty acids). The best source is cold-pressed flax seed oil and primrose oil. Other good sources are fish oil, canola oil,

Anyone who desires to be proactive with their health needs to take this level of supplementation. Regular, off-the-shelf multivitamins have not been shown in medical literature to produce a significant health benefit. The main reason is the fact that they are usually providing their nutrients at the traditional RDA level. The level of supplementation that I have recommended has been shown in medical literature to be effective and safe in properly nourishing your cells at an optimal level, so what are the health benefits that my patients receive when they start the supplementation program I have just recommended?

1. They decrease their risk of cardiovascular disease (heart attack, stroke, and hardening of the arteries in general) because they make LDL cholesterol less vulnerable to being oxidized. Also, their homocysteine level decreases substantially, allowing this risk factor to be eliminated.
2. They decrease risk of developing cancer.
3. They improve their own immune system.
4. They decrease their risk of age-related cataract formation and the development of age-related macular degeneration.
5. Hopefully, they decrease their risk of Alzheimer's dementia, Parkinson's disease, rheumatoid arthritis, osteoarthritis, Crohn's disease, and all the other degenerative diseases that we are now discovering are caused by oxidative stress.
6. Asthma and the progression of emphysema may improve for the better.
7. Hopefully, we'll see that they even decrease their risk of the development of diabetes.
8. The progression of osteoporosis slows and possibly is even prevented.

Does this mean I am offering a treatment for these diseases? No. Just as patients who have a moderate exercise program will receive a health benefit, patients who start a good quality nutritional supplement program will receive a health benefit. This is NOT alternative medicine. It is main-line, traditional, preventative medicine that is based on our medical literature. I am simply building up my patients' own antioxidant defense systems and their own immune system. The body is our best defense against the development of chronic degenerative disease. We just need to have it working at its optimal level.

WHAT IF I ALREADY HAVE A CHRONIC DEGENERATIVE DISEASE?

There is no argument that it is much easier to maintain your health than it is to regain it after you have lost it. Most people assume that they will always have good health. Very few patients plan on losing their health. As a physician, I spend much of my time consulting with patients who have lost their health. I may be telling them that they have coronary artery disease, or have just developed diabetes, or even that they have cancer. Once you have developed a chronic degenerative disease, things are not totally lost. Aggressive nutritional supplementation has allowed several of my patients to take back control of their health. They are not cured of their disease, but they do have significant improvement in their health.

I begin by placing my patients with a chronic degenerative disease on the same basic supplement program that I outlined in Table 1. However, I add some of the more potent antioxidants to their regimen. One of the best is proanthocyanidins, which I believe are the most potent antioxidants known today. They are derived primarily from either pine bark or grape seeds. Personally, I believe the grape seed extracts are more potent. They have some characteristics that make them ideal for individuals who are already suffering from chronic degenerative diseases. They are several times more potent that vitamin E and vitamin C as antioxidants. They readily cross over into the fluid around the brain and nerves. They also have anti-inflammatory properties and work synergistically with all the other antioxidants. I may also add higher levels of Coenzyme Q10 to my patients with cardiomyopathy or cancer.

Now that we are beginning to appreciate the role of oxidative stress in chronic degenerative diseases, everyone will be trying to find the most potent antioxidants that they can. Remember: the best results are obtained when good levels of several antioxidants are used to create a synergistic effect, rather than relying on massive doses of a single antioxidant. So if you are going to use some of these more potent antioxidants, make sure that you are adding them to a complete, balanced, nutritional program.

I would like to add just a word of caution. I believe we may see some studies which will show that using a single antioxidant alone in massive doses may actually cause it to become a prooxidant (actually create more free radicals).

That is another reason why I believe we need to add these more potent antioxidants to a complete, balanced, nutritional-supplement program and not rely on just one nutrient. I have been able to achieve tremendous results in my patients by applying these principles.

HOW DO YOU CHOOSE A QUALITY NUTRITIONAL SUPPLEMENT?

There is no federal regulation of the vitamin supplement market. The Dietary Supplement Health and Education Act of 1994 pretty much left the nutritional supplement market unregulated. The government treats these supplements as food and not as over-the-counter drugs.

When I did not believe in taking supplements, I advised my patients who wanted to take supplements to buy the cheapest ones. My attitude has since changed. There is a difference in supplements and in the way they are manufactured. I advise my patients to get the best quality supplements that they can afford. I realize that this can be a significant economic decision for most people. Everyone needs to assess the importance of their health and what value they place on it. I look at nutritional supplements as my health insurance. I already have death insurance—which is my life insurance. I want to do everything that I possibly can to protect my health. Whatever life the Lord allows me to have, I want to live as healthy as possible. Good health is definitely a blessing. Once you lose your health, no amount of money that you have or are willing to spend can usually restore it.

If you have ever walked into a health food store and looked at the number of supplements available today, you know it is overwhelming. My purpose in writing this book is not to recommend a particular manufacturing company. Therefore, I will share some basic principles to consider when choosing a supplement.

There are companies now that are putting many of these antioxidants and their supporting nutrients together. Unless you like taking a lot of pills, this would be a good start. There is no way you are going to get the amount of supplementation I have recommended into one tablet. So a one-a-day multivitamin simply will not do. Minerals are also better when they are in a balanced mineral formula rather than as isolated minerals. Minerals are also very hard to absorb; therefore, I recommend chelated minerals, which have been shown in medical literature to be most easily absorbed.

Furthermore, there is significant interaction between various minerals, and by taking them separately you may actually create more problems. For example, the body needs copper to absorb iron. However, if we take in just a little too much zinc, it blocks the absorption of copper, which decreases the absorption of iron, which could lead to iron-deficiency anemia and so forth.

The supplement you choose needs to be able to dissolve or you won't absorb the nutrients. The November 1997 newsletter from Tufts University looked at a study from the University of Maryland where nine different prescription, prenatal vitamins were studied just to see if they dissolved. It was discovered that only three of the nine prescribed prenatal vitamins even dissolved. Ten more prenatal vitamins were studied and two failed miserably. Only those vitamins that had followed U.S. Pharmacopoeia (USP) standards completely dissolved. Choosing companies that submit to the USP standards of dissolution is clearly a step in the right direction.

My best advice in choosing a particular nutritional company is to research the company's Internet web site or actually call the company. Find out if they manufacture their supplements in a FDA-registered manufacturing facility. Ask them or find out if they follow good manufacturing practices (GMP). It would be better yet if they followed GMP for pharmaceuticals. This means that they produce a nutritional product with the same quality as if they were making a brand-name drug. Even though the government does not require this, some companies choose to do it because they want to create a quality, pharmaceutical-grade product. Some companies follow the GMP guidelines for foods. These guidelines are much less strict than the GMP guidelines for pharmaceuticals, but they are better than no accountability at all.

Quality nutritional companies will put in the actual amounts of their compounds and will give full disclosure of all their ingredients. Also, they usually have an expiration date, and their full address (not a post office box) is on the bottle.

If you live in Canada, you can look for a drug identification number (DIN) on the bottle. This assures you that the Canadian government has certified the product. If you live in Australia, you can look for an AUSTL listing on the bottle. This tells you that the Australian government has evaluated it.

BIONUTRITION

Conclusion

There are many physicians who are beginning to realize the value of recommending nutritional supplements to their patients. There is no way you can avoid reading about supplements and their relation to our health in main-line medical literature. So why are so many physicians against their patients taking nutritional supplements?

Practicing physicians face many obstacles when considering recommending supplements to their patients. First and foremost, they must overcome a bias against supplements that began back in medical school. The peer pressure from other physicians is no small obstacle, either. Their basic lack of knowledge in the field of nutritional science is not helpful. Physicians become very concerned when their patients are using supplements as an alternative therapy to traditional medical care. Most physicians, though, simply do not believe that the medical evidence is strong enough to begin recommending supplements. If they did, there wouldn't be any reason for me to write this book.

As I write this final chapter, I noted a study that illustrates the difficulty physicians face in this ever-growing field of nutritional supplementation. This is the lead article in the March 19, 1998, issue of the New England Journal of Medicine. The title of the article is "Hypovitaminosis D in Medical Patients."

Melissa K. Thomas, MD, et al, studied 290 consecutive patients who entered the general medical wards at Massachusetts General Hospital. They evaluated these patients for vitamin D deficiency. They eliminated patients who were from nursing homes or who had significant chronic diseases. They divided their group to account for seasonal sun exposure. They found that 57 percent of these patients had significant vitamin D deficiencies. They used the criteria that having a vitamin D level below 15 ng per milliliter was insufficient to maintain adequate bone health.

However, the authors noted that many researchers have shown that a level of 30 ng per milliliter is needed to maintain adequate bone health. When this level was applied to their findings, 93 percent of the patients had a vitamin D deficiency. Patients who took multivitamins (RDA levels of vitamin D) showed absolutely no benefit. Patients needed to take much higher levels of vitamin D supplementation (near 800 IU) in order to provide adequate vitamin D levels. These authors concluded that because of the potential adverse effects of vitamin D deficiency on the skeleton and other organ systems, widespread screening for vitamin D deficiency or routine vitamin D supplementation should be considered.

Now, none of these patients had rickets. This is the acute deficiency disease people get when they have a severe deficiency of vitamin D. This is why the RDA levels of nutrients were established, so that we could avoid these acute deficiency diseases. So the deficiencies mentioned in this study are concerned about optimal levels of vitamin D. In order to obtain an optimal level of vitamin D so that our bodies can function at their peak level, we may need 800 IU of vitamin D in supplementation. This is BIONUTRITION. Simply put, we want to avoid osteoporosis and its devastating effects on our health. The RDA of vitamin D for adults older than 25 years of age is 200 IU. A multiple vitamin will not provide you with 800 IU. So a physician who appreciates what this study means will recommend that his or her patients start taking vitamin D supplements.

As a physician, when you begin to understand oxidative stress as it relates to our health, antioxidants take on a new meaning. In order to prevent oxidative stress and repair the damage it does to the body, we need to have adequate levels of natural antioxidants available. I personally do not believe that pharmaceutical drugs hold the answer to many of the health problems that we are presently facing. Antioxidants and phytochemicals (natural plant nutrients) that have potent antioxidant properties have more promise. Now, don't sell the pharmaceutical companies short. They understand the strong potential that antioxidants have to offer and are now beginning to develop synthetic antioxidants as a means to develop newer drugs. Two drugs that have been shown to have synthetic antioxidant properties were released in the past year, Rezulin for diabetes and Coreg for congestive heart failure. Natural antioxidants are not only more effective but also safer and less expensive. However, the drug companies will certainly try to take advantage of the growing body of medical evidence presented in this book.

Physicians and lay people alike must begin looking at nutritional supplements as a way to enhance the natural metabolic activities that the body must perform. We need all these essential nutrients in supplementation. By recommending a complete, balanced, nutritional-supplement program, it makes it simple for the practicing physician. Then when he or she reads a study like the one on vitamin D deficiency in the New England Journal of Medicine, they can simply say to themselves, "I am glad that I have already been recommending this level of supplementation to my patients."

I have presented a significant amount of information regarding supplementation found in the current medical literature. As impressive as these studies are, they are not the main reason I wrote this book. The results that I have seen in my patients since I began to recommend nutritional supplements have been nothing short of amazing. I am helping patients in ways that I never dreamed possible in the past. My passionate search within medical literature was an attempt to try to explain the results I was witnessing in my practice. My mission is now to share this knowledge with my fellow physicians so that they, in turn, will be able to help their patients. I pray that this information has helped you and given you an insight into how you can better protect your own health.

Remember the principles you have learned in this book. This will be a dynamic, changing field of medicine. The amounts and levels of supplementation will be changing as we gain more knowledge. There will be new studies appearing frequently in our medical journals as well as in the lay media. Newer and more potent natural antioxidants will be discovered. I believe that most of the great advances in medicine over the next 20 to 30 years will come in the field of nutritional science.

You are welcome to learn more about what I specifically recommend to my patients by searching my web site at www.raystrand.com. Thank you for the time you spent reading this book. I hope your health benefits.

References

Chapter 2

1. Kelvin Davies. "Oxidative stress, the paradox of aerobic life." Biochemical Society Symposia 61 (1995): 1-31.
2. Anthony Diplock. "Antioxidant nutrients and disease prevention: an overview." American Journal of Clinical Nutrition 53, no. 1 (January 1991 [supplement]): 189S-93S.
3. Paolo Di Mascio, Michael Murphy, and Helmut Sies. "Antioxidant defense systems: The role of carotenoids, tocopherols, thiols." American Journal of Clinical Nutrition 53 (1991): 194S-200S.
4. Peter Moller, Hakan Wallin, and Lizbeth Knudsen. "Oxidative stress associated with exercise, psychological stress and life-style factors." Chemico-Biological Interactions 102, no. 1 (September 27, 1996): 17-36.
5. Kenneth Cooper, MD. "The Antioxidant Revolution." Nashville, TN: Thomas Nelson Publishers, 1994

Chapter 3

1. Daniel Steinberg, MD; Sampath Parthasarathy, Ph.D.; Thomas Carew, Ph. D, et al. "Beyond cholesterol: Modifications of low-density lipoprotein that increase its atherogenicity." New England Journal of Medicine 320, no. 14 (April 16, 1989): 915-924.
2. Marco Diaz, MD; Balz Frei, Ph.D.; Joseph Vita, MD; and John Keaney, Jr., MD. "Antioxidants and atherosclerotic heart disease." New England Journal of Medicine 337, no. 6 (August 7, 1997): 408-416.
3. Meir J. Stampfer, MD; Charles H. Hennekens, MD; et al. "Vitamin E consumption and the risk of coronary disease in women." New England Journal of Medicine 328 (May 20, 1993): 1444-1449.
4. Jan Regnström, Jan Nilsson, et al. "Susceptibility to low-density lipoprotein oxidation and coronary atherosclerosis in men." Lancet 339 (May 16, 1992): 1183-1186.
5. Daniel Steinberg, MD, Ph.D. "Antioxidants in the prevention of human atherosclerosis." Summary of the proceedings of a National Heart, Lung, and Blood Institute workshop; September 5-6, 1991 Bethesda, Maryland. Circulation 85 (1992): 62337-62347.
6. Hermann Esterbauer, et al. "Role of vitamin E in preventing the oxidation of low-density lipoprotein." The American Journal of Clinical Nutrition 53 (1991): 312S-321S.
7. Dexter L. Morris, Ph.D., MD; Steven Kritchevsky, Ph. D.; and C. E. Davis, Ph.D. "Serum carotenoids and coronary heart disease." JAMA 272, no. 18 (November 9, 1994): 1439-1441.
8. R. N. Acheson, and D.R.R. Williams. "Does consumption of fruits and vegetables protect against stroke?" Lancet 1 (1993): 1191-1193.
9. B. K. Armstrong, J. L. Mann, et al. "Commodity consumption and ischemic heart disease mortality, with specific reference to dietary practices." Journal of Chronic Disease 36 (1975): 673-677.
10. K. F. Gey, and P. Puska. "Plasma vitamins E and A inversely correlated to mortality ischemic heart disease in cross-cultural epidemiology." Annals New York Academy of Science 570 (1989): 254-282.
11. A. J. Verlangieri, J. C. Kapeghian, et al. "Fruit and vegetable consumption and cardiovascular disease mortality." Medical Hypotheses 16 (1985): 7-15.
12. R. A. Riemersma, M. Oliver, et al. "Plasma antioxidants and coronary heart disease: Vitamin C and E and selenium." European Journal of Clinical Nutrition 44 (1990): 143-150.
13. J. Ramirez, and N. C. Flowers. "Leukocyte ascorbic acid and its relationship to coronary heart disease in man." American Journal of Clinical Nutrition 33 (1980): 2079-2087.
14. J. E. Manson, M. J. Stampfer, et al. "A perspective study of antioxidant vitamins and incidence of coronary heart disease in women." Circulation 84 (1991 [supplement II]): 4.
15. J. E. Manson, M. J. Stampfer, et al. "A perspective study of vitamin C and incidence of coronary heart disease in women." Circulation 85 (1992): 3,865.

16. M. J. Stampfer, J. E. Manson, et al. "A perspective study of vitamin E supplementation and risk of coronary disease in women." Circulation 86 (1992 [supplement I]): 1847.

17. E. B. Rimm, A. Ascherio, et al. "Vitamin E supplementation and risk of coronary heart disease among men." Circulation 86 (1992 [supplement I]): 1848.

18. J. E. Engstrom, L. E. Kenin, M. A. Klein. "Vitamin C intake and mortality among a sample of the United States population." Epidemiology 3 (1992): 194-202.

19. Alpha-tocopherol, beta-carotene cancer prevention study group. "The effect of vitamin E and beta-carotene on the incidence of lung cancer and other cancers in male smokers." New England Journal of Medicine 330 (1994):1029-1035.

20. Howard N. Hodis, MD; et al. "Serial coronary angiographic evidence that antioxidant vitamin intake reduces progression of coronary artery atherosclerosis." JAMA 273, no. 23 (1995): 1849-1854.

21. Dexter L. Morris, Ph.D., MD; Steven B. Kritchevsky, Ph.D.; and C. E. Davis, Ph,D. "Serum carotenoids and coronary heart disease." JAMA 272, no. 18 (November 9, 1994): 1439-1441.

22. Nigel G. Stephens, et al. "Randomised controlled trial of vitamin E and patients with coronary disease: Cambridge Heart Antioxidant Study (CHAOS)." Lancet 347 (March 23, 1996): 781-786.

23. Marco N. Diaz, MD, et al. "Antioxidants and atherosclerotic heart disease." New England Journal of Medicine 337 (August 7, 1997): 408-416.

Chapter 4

1. Michelle Stacey. "The fall and rise of Kilmer McClay." New York Times Magazine (August 10, 1997): 26-29.

2. M. J. Stampfer, M. R. Malinow, W. C. Willett, et al. "A perspective study of plasma homocysteine and risk of myocardial infarction." U.S. Physicians Journal of the American Medical Association 268 (1992): 877-881.

3. R. Ross, Ph.D., and J. A. Glomset, MD. "The pathogenesis of atherosclerosis." New England Journal of Medicine 295, no. 7 (1996): 369-375.

4. Jacob Selhub, Ph.D., P. F. Jacques, et al. "Association between plasma homocysteine concentrations and extracranial carotid artery stenosis." New England Journal of Medicine 332, no. 5 (February 2, 1995): 286-291.

5. E. Arnesen, H. Refsum, K. H. Bonaa, et al. "Serum total homocysteine and coronary heart disease." International Journal of Epidemiology 24 (1995):704-709.

6. C. J. Boushey, S. A. Beresford, G. S. Omen, A. G. Motulsky. "A quantitative assessment of plasma homocysteine as a risk factor for vascular disease." JAMA 274 (1995):1049-1057.

7. D. S. Rosenblatt. "Inherited disorders of folate transport and metabolism." In The Metabolic Basis of Inherited Disease, 6th ed. C. R. Scriver, A. L. Beaudet, W. S. Sly, and D. Valle, eds. New York: McGraw-Hill, 1989, pp. 2049-2064.

8. H. J. Naurath, E. Joosten, R. Riezler, et al. "Effects of vitamin B-12, folate, and vitamin B-6 supplements in elderly with normal serum vitamin concentrations." Lancet 346 (1995): 85-89.

9. G. J. Cuskelly, H. McNulty, J. M. Scott. "Effect of increasing dietary folate on red-cell folate: Implications for prevention of neural tube defects." Lancet 347 (March 9, 1996): 657-659.

10. J. E. Brown, Ph.D., D. R. Jacobs, Jr., Ph.D., et al. "Predictors of red-cell folate level in women attempting pregnancy." JAMA 277, no. 6 (February 19, 1997): 548-552.

11. M.R. Malinow, et al. "Reduction of plasma homocysteine levels by breakfast cereal fortified with folic acid in patients with coronary artery disease." New England Journal of Medicine 338, no. 15 (April 9, 1998): 1009-1015.

12. Russell Ross, Ph. D. "Atherosclerosis – An Inflammatory Disease." New England Journal of Medicine 340, no. 2 (January 14,1999): 115-123

Chapter 5

1. G. P . Littarru, S. Lippa, et al. "Metabolic and diagnostic implications of blood CoQ10 levels." In: Biomedical and Clinical Aspects of Coenzyme Q10, vol. 6. K. Folkers, T. Yamagami, G. P. Littarru, eds.: Elsevier, Amsterdam, 1991, pp. 167-178.

2. E. Baggio, R. Gandini, et al. "Italian multi-center study on the safety and efficacy of Coenzyme Q10 as adjunctive therapy in heart failure." Molecular Aspects of Medicine 15 (1994 [supplement]): S287-S294.

3. P. H. Langsjoen, K. Folkers, et al. "Effective and safe therapy with Coenzyme Q10 for cardiomyopathy." Klinische Wochenschrift 66, no. 13 (July 1, 1988): 583-590.

4. P. H. Langsjoen, K. Folkers, et al. "Pronounced increase of survival in patients with cardiomyopathy when treated with Coenzyme Q10 and conventional therapy." International Journal of Tissue Reactions 12, no. 3 (1990):163-168.

5. P. H. Langsjoen, and K. Folkers. "A six-year clinical study of therapy of cardiomyopathy with Coenzyme Q10." International Journal of Tissue Reactions 12, no. 3 (1990):169-171.

6. U. Manzoli, E. Rossi, et al. "Coenzyme Q10 and dilated cardiomyopathy." Int J Tissue React 12, no. 3 (1990) :173-178.

7. A. Davini, F. Cellerini, and P. L. Topi. "Coenzyme Q10: Contractile dysfunction of the myocardial cell and metabolic therapy." Minerva Cardioangiologica 40, no. 11 (November 1992): 449-453.

8. S. A. Mortensen. "Perspectives on therapy of cardiovascular diseases with Coenzyme Q10." Clinical Investigation 71 (1993 [supplement VIII]): S116-S123.

9. H. Langsjoen, P. Langsjoen, et al. "Usefulness of Coenzyme Q10 in clinical cardiology: A long-term study." Molecular Aspects of Medicine 15 (1994 [supplement]): S165-S175.

10. K. Folkers, P. Langsjoen, P. H. Langsjoen. "Therapy with Coenzyme Q10 of patients with heart failure who are eligible or ineligible for a transplant." Biochemical and Biophysical Research Communications 182, no. 1 (January 15, 1992): 247-253.

Chapter 6

1. A. T. Diplok. "Antioxidant nutrients and disease prevention: An overview." American Journal of Nutrition 53 (1991): 189S-193S.

2. Calvin Davies. "Oxidative stress: The paradox of aerobic life." Biochem Soc Symp 61 (1995): 1-31.

3. Tom Paulson. "Seattle biochemist challenging cancer theories." Seattle Post-Intelligencer (November 26, 1996): 1.

4. Rebecca Voelker. "Ames agrees with mom's advice: Eat your fruits and vegetables." JAMA 273, no. 14 (April 12, 1995):1077-1078.

5. M. Kodama, Kanekom, et al. "Free radical chemistry of cigarette smoke and its implication in human cancer." Anti-cancer Research 17, no. 1A (January/February 1997): 433-437.

6. Peter Moller, H. Wallin, and L. Knudsen. "Oxidative stress associated with exercise, psychological stress, and life-style factors." Chemico-Biological Interactions 102 (1996): 17-36.

7. S. J. Duthie, M. A. Aiguo, M. A. Ross, and A. R. Collins. "Antioxidant supplementation decreases oxidative DNA damage in human lymphocytes." Cancer Research 15, no. 56(6) (March 1996): 1291-1295.

8. A. Hartmann, A. M. Niess, et al. "Vitamin E prevents exercise-induced DNA damage." Mutation Research 348, no. 4 (April 1995): 195-202.

9. L. C. Clark, et al. "Effects of selenium supplementation for cancer prevention in patients with carcinoma of the skin. A randomized controlled trial. Nutritional Prevention of Cancer Study Group." JAMA 276, no. 24 (1996): 1957-1963

10. B. A. Lashner, et al. "The effect of folic acid supplementation on the risk of cancer or dysplasia in ulcerative colitis." Gastroenterology 112, no. 1 (January 1997): 29-32.

11. E. W. Flagg, R. J. Coates, and R. S. Greenberg. "Epidemiologic studies of antioxidants in cancer in humans." Journal of the American College of Nutrition 14, no. 5 (October 1995): 419-427.

BIONUTRITION

12. G. Shklar, J. Schwartz, et al. "The effectiveness of a mixture of beta-carotene, alpha-tocopherol, glutathione and ascorbic acid for cancer prevention." Nutrition and Cancer 20, no. 2 (1993): 145-151.

13. W. L. Stone, A. M. Papas. "Tocopherols and the etiology of colon cancer." Journal of the National Cancer Institute 89, no. 14 (July 16, 1997): 1006-1014.

14. M. Lipkin, and H. Newark. "Effect of added dietary calcium on colonic epithelial-cell proliferation in subjects at high risk for familial colonic cancer." New England Journal of Medicine 313, no. 22 (November 28, 1985): 1381-1384.

15. P. Knekt, R. Jarvinen, et al. "Dietary flavanoids and the risk of lung cancer and other malignant neoplasms." American Journal of Epidemiology 146, no. 3 (August 1, 1997): 223-230.

16. K. Folkers, A. Osterborg, et al. "Activities of vitamin CoQ10 in animal models and a serious deficiency in patients with cancer." Biochemical and Biophysical Research Communications 234, no. 2 (May 19, 1997): 296-299.

17. D. Jiao, T. J. Smith, et al. "Chemopreventive activity of thiol conjugates of isothiocyanates for lung tumorigenesis." Carcinogenesis 18, no. 11 (November 1997): 2143-2147.

18. H. S. Garewal, MD, Ph.D.; S. Schantz, MD. "Emerging role of beta-carotene and antioxidant nutrients in prevention of oral cancer." Archives Otolaryngol Head Neck Surgery 212 (February 1995): 141-144.

19. G. Shklar, et al. "The effectiveness of a mixture of beta-carotene, alpha-tochopherol, glutathione, and ascorbic acid for cancer prevention." Nutrition and Cancer (1993); 20; 145-151.

20. G. E. Kaugars, S. Silverman, Jr., et al. "A clinical trial of antioxidant supplements in the treatment of oral leukaplakia." Oral Surgery Oral Medicine Oral Pathology 78, no. 4 (October 1994): 462-468.

21. C. O. Enwonwu, and V. I. Meeks. "Bionutriton and oral cancer in humans." Critical Reviews in Oral Biology and Medicine 6, no. 1 (1995): 5-17.

22. H. Garewal. "Antioxidants and oral cancer prevention." American Journal of Clinical Nutrition 62 (December 1995 [supplement VI]): 1410S-1416S.

23. S. L. Romney, et al. "Nutrient antioxidants in the pathogenesis and prevention of cervical dysplasia and cancer." J Scell Biochem Suppl 23 (1995): 96-103.

24. F. L. Meyskens, Jr., and A. Manetta. "Prevention of cervical intraepithelial neoplasia and cervical cancer." American Journal of Clinical Nutrition 62, no. 6 (December 1995 [supplement]): 1417S-1419S.

25. Y. Muto, et al. "Growth retardation in human cervical dysplasia-derived cell lines by beta-carotene through down-regulation of epidermal growth factor receptor." American Journal of Clinical Nutrition 62 (December 1995 [supplement VI]): 1535S-1540S.

26. R. Chinery, J. A. Brokman, et al. "Antioxidants enhance the cytotoxicity of chemotherapeutic agents in colorectal cancer." Natural Medicine 3, no. 11 (November 1997): 1233-1241.

27. K. Lockwood, S. Moesgaard, et al. "Progress in therapy of breast cancer with vitamin CoQ10 and the regression of metastasis." Biochemical and Biophysical Research Communications 212, no. 1 (July 6, 1995):172-177.

28. K. Jaakkola, P. Lahteenmaki, et al. "Treatment with antioxidant other nutrients in combination with chemotherapy and irradiation in patients with small cell lung cancer." Anti-cancer Research 12 (1992): 599-606.

29. N. T. Telang, M. Katdare, et al. "Inhibition and proliferation in modulation of estrodial metabolism: Novel mechanisms for breast cancer prevention by the phytochemical Indole-3-carbinol." Proc Soc Exp Biol Med 216, no. 2 (November 1997): 246-252.

30. K. Lockwood, S. Moesgaard, and K. Folkers. "Partial and complete regression of breast cancer in patients in relation to dosage of Coenzyme Q10." Biochemical and Biophysical Research Communications 199, no. 3 (March 30, 1994): 1504-1508.

Chapter 7

1. G. E. Marak, et al. "Free radicals and antioxidants in the pathogenesis of eye diseases." Advances in Experimental Medicine and Biology 264 (1990): 513-527.

2. S. J. Stohs. "The role of free radicals in toxicity and disease." Journal of Basic and Clinical Physiology and Pharmacology 6 (1995): 3-4, 205-228.

3. P. Knekt, et al. "Serum antioxidant vitamins and risk of cataract". British Medical Journal 305 (1992): 1392-1394.

4. J. M. Robertson, et al. "Vitamin E intake and risk of cataracts in humans." Annals of the New York Academy of Science 570 (1989): 372-382.

5. H. Heseker. "Antioxidative vitamins and cataracts in the elderly". Zeitschrift Fur Ernahrungswissenschaft 34, no. 3 (September 1995): 167-176.

6. I. Maitra, et al. "Alpha-lipoic acid prevents buthionine sulfoximine-induced cataract formation in newborn rats". Free Radical Biology and Medicine 18, no. 4 (1995): 823-829.

7. W. G. Christen, et al. "Antioxidants and age-related eye disease current and future perspectives." Annals of Epidemiology 6 (1996): 60-66.

8. A. M. Vanderhagen, et al. "Free radicals and antioxidant supplementation: A review of their roles in age-related macular degeneration." Journal of the American Optometry Association 1993 64, no. 12 (December 1993): 871-878.

9. J. M. Seddon, et al. "Dietary carotenoids, vitamins A, C, and E, and advanced age-related macular degeneration." Eye disease case-control study group. JAMA 272, no. 18 (November 9, 1994): 1413-1420.

10. N. Ishihara, et al. "Antioxidants and angiogenetic factor associated with age-related macular degeneration" Nippon Ganka Gakkai Zasshi 101, no. 3 (1997): 248-251.

11. S. Richer. "Multicenter ophthalmic and nutritional age-related macular degeneration study. Part 1: design, subjects and procedures." Journal of the American Optometry Association 67, no. 1 (January 1996): 12-29.

12. P. S. Bernstein, et al. "Retinal tubulin binds macular carotenoids". Investigative Ophthalmology and Visual Science 38, no. 1 (January 1997): 167-175.

13. J. T. Landrum, et al. "A one-year study of macular pigment: The effect of 140 days of a lutein supplement." Experimental Research 65, no. 1 (July 1997): 57-62.

14. R. W. Young. "Solar radiation and age-related macular degeneration." Survey of Ophthalmology 23, (1988): 252-269.

15. D. M. Snodderly "Evidence for protection against age-related macular degeneration by carotenoids and antioxidant vitamins." American Journal of Clinical Nutrition 62 (December 1995 [supplement 6]): 1448S-1461S.

Chapter 8

1. P. H. Evans "Free radicals and brain metabolism and pathology". British Medical Bulletin 49, no. 3 (July 1993): 577-587.

2. Joseph Knight, MD "Reactive oxygen species in the neurodegenerative disorders." Annals of Clinical and Laboratory Science 27, no.1 (November 3, 1996): 11-25 Alzheimer's Dementia

3. D. B. Carr, MD, et al. "Current concepts in the pathogenesis of Alzheimer's disease." American Journal of Medicine 103, no. 3A (September 22, 1997): 3S-10S.

4. M. A. Smith, and G. Perry. "Free radical damage, iron, and Alzheimer's disease." Journal of the Neurological Sciences 134 (1995 [supplement]): 92-94.

5. M. Sano, C. Ernesto, et al. "A controlled trial of selegiline, alpha-tocopheral, or both as treatment for Alzheimer's disease." New England Journal of Medicine 336, no. 17 (April 24, 1997): 1216-1222.

6. P. H. Evans, et al. "Oxidative damage and Alzheimer's dementia, and the potential etiopathogenic role of aluminosilicates, microglia and micronutrient interactions." Free Radicals and Aging 1992, ed. by I. Emmerit & B. Chance: 178-189. Parkinson's Disease

7. Stanley Fahn. "An open trial of high-dosage antioxidants in early Parkinson's disease." American Journal of Clinical Nutrition 53 (1991): 380S-382S.

8. D. Offen, et al. "Prevention of dopamine-induced cell death by thiol antioxidants: Possible implications for treatment of Parkinson's disease." Experimental Neurology 141, no. 1 (September 1996): 32-39.

9. M. Ebadi, et al. "Oxidative stress and antioxidant therapy in Parkinson's disease." Progress in Neurobiology 48, no. 1 (January 1996): 1-19.

10. The Parkinson Study Group. "Effects of tocopherol and deprenyl on the progression of disability in early Parkinson's disease." New England Journal of Medicine 328, no. 3 (January 21, 1993): 176-183. Multiple Sclerosis

11. S. M. LeVine "The role of reactive oxygen species in the pathogenesis of multiple sclerosis". Medical Hypotheses 39, no. 3 (November 1992):271-274.

12. Calabrese V, et al. "Changes in cerebral spinal fluid levels of malondialdehyde and glutathione reductase activity in multiple sclerosis." International Journal of Clinical Pharmacology and Laboratory Research 14, no. 4 (1994): 119-123.

13. Toshniwal PK, Zarling ZJ. "Evidence for increased lipid perioxidation in multiple sclerosis." Neurochemical Research 17, no. 2 (February 1992): 205-207.

14. L. Bow , T. M. Dawson, et al. "Induction of nitric oxide synthesis in demyelinating regions of multiple sclerosis brains." Annals of Neurology 36, no. 5 (November 1994): 778-786.

15. Beal FM. "Mitochondria, free radicals and neurodegeneration." Current Opinion in Neurobiology 6 (1996): 661-666. Amyotrophic Lateral Sclerosis

16. C. W. Aolanow, and G. W. Arendash "Metals and free radicals in neurodegeneration". Current Opinion in Neurology 7, no. 6 (December 1994): 548-558.

17. P. I. Oteiza, et al. "Evaluation of antioxidants protein and lipid oxidation products and blood from sporadic amyotrophic lateral sclerosis." Neurochemical Research 44, no. 4 (April 1997): 535-9.

18. G. D. Ghadge, et al. "Mutant superoxide dismutase-1-linked familial amyotrophic lateral sclerosis: Molecular mechanisms of neuronal death and protection." Journal of Neurological Science 17, no. 22 (November 15, 1997): 8756-8766.

19. A. Vyth, et al. "Survival in patients with amyotrophic lateral sclerosis, treated with an array of antioxidants." Journal of Neurological Science 139 (August 1996 [supplement]): 99-103.

20. F. Terro, et al. "Antioxidant drugs block in vitro the neurotoxicity of CSF from patients with amyotrophic later sclerosis." Neurology Report 7, no. 12 (August 12, 1996): 1970-1972. Inflammatory Bowel Disease

21. T. P. Mulder, et al. "Effect of oral zinc supplementation on metallothionein and superoxide dismutase concentrations in patients with inflammatory bowel disease." Journal of Gastroenterol Hepatology 9, no. 5 (September-October 1994): 472-477.

22. L. Lih-Brody, et al. "Increased oxidative stress in decreased antioxidant defenses in mucosa of inflammatory bowel disease." Digestive Diseases and Science 41, no. 10 (October 1996); 2078-2086.

23. A. Burke, et al. "Nutrition and ulcerative colitis." Baillieres Clinical Gastroenterology 11, no. 1 (March 1997): 153-174.

24. I. Beno, et al. "Ulcerative colitis: Activity of antioxidant enzymes of the colonic mucosa." Presse Med 26, no. 31 (October 18, 1997): 1474-1477.

25. E. J. Hoffenberg, et al. "Circulating antioxidant concentration in children with inflammatory bowel disease." American Journal of Clinical Nutrition 65, no. 5 (May 1997): 1482-1488.

26. T. Iantomasi, et al. "Glutathione metabolism in Crohn's disease." Biochemical Medicine and Metabolic Biology 53, no. 2 (December 1994): 87-91.

27. G. D. Buffinton, and W. F. Doe. "Depleted mucosal antioxidant status in inflammatory bowel disease." Free Radical Research 22, no. 2 (February 1995): 131-143.

28. S. J. McKenzie, et al. "Evidence of oxidant-induced injury to epithelial cells during inflammatory bowel disease." Journal of Clinical Investigation 98, no. 1 July 1, 1996): 136-141.

29. G. D. Buffinton, and W. F. Doe. "Depleted mecosal antioxidant defenses in inflammatory bowel disease." Free Radical Biology and Medicine 19, no. 6 (December 1995): 911-918. Pulmonary Disease

30. I. Rahman, et al. "Systemic oxidative stress in asthma, COPD, and smokers." American Journal of Respiratory Critical Care Medicine 154 (1996): 1055-1060.

31. Z. Novak, et al. "Examination of the role of oxygen free radicals in bronchial asthma in childhood." Clinica Chimica Acta 201, no. 3 (September 30 1991): 247-251.

32. G. E. Hatch "Asthma, inhaled oxidants, and dietary antioxidants." American Journal of Clinical Nutrition 61 (1995 [supplement]): 625S-630S.

33. P. J. Barnes. "Reactive oxygen species and airway inflammation." Free Radical Biology in Medicine 9 (1990): 235-243. Arthritis

34. Y. Henrotin, et al. "Active oxygen species, articular inflammation and cartilage damage". EXS-Free Radicals and Aging 62 (1992): 308-322.

35. R. Miesel, et al. "Enhanced mitochondrial radical production in patients with rheumatoid arthritis correlates with elevated levels of tumor necrosis factor alpha in plasma." Free Radical Research 25, no. 2 (August 1996): 161-169.

36. P. Mary, et al. "Oxidative damage to lipids within the inflamed human joint provides evidence of radical-mediated hypoxic-reperfusion injury." American Journal of Clinical Nutrition 53 (1991): 362S-369S.

37. G. W. Comstock, et al. "Serum concentrations of alpha-tocopherol, beta-carotene, and retinol preceding the diagnosis of rheumatoid arthritis and systemic lupus erythematosis." Annals of Rheumatic Diseases 56, no. 5 (May 1997): 323-325.

38. T. E. McAlindon, et al. "Relation of dietary intake and serum levels of vitamin D to progression of osteoarthritis of the knee among participants in the Framingham Study". Annals of Internal Medicine 125, no. 5 (September 1, 1996): 353-359.

39. D. Singh, et al. "Electron spin resonance spectroscopic demonstration of the generation of reactive oxygen species by diseased human synovial tissue following ex vivo hypoxia-reoxygenation." Annals of Rheumatoid Disease 54, no. 2 (February 1995): 94-99.

40. T. E. McAlindon, et al. "Do antioxidant micronutrients protect against the development and progression of osteoarthitis." Arthritis and Rheumatism 39, no. 4 (April 1996): 648-656.

41. L. Flohé. "Superoxide dismutase for therapeutic use: Clinical experience, dead end and hopes." Molecular and Cellular Biochemistry 84 (1998): 123-131.

42. K. H. Schmidt, and W. Bayer. "Efficacy of vitamin E as a drug in inflammatory joint disease." Antioxidants in Therapy and Preventative Medicine. I. Emerit, et al., eds. New York: Plenum Press, 1990, pp. 147-150.

43. H. M. Meltzer, et al. "Selenium supplementation in rheumatics." Abstracts of the Proceedings of Metabolisms of trace elements related to human disease. Loen, Norway. Symposium. (1985):36.

Chapter 9

1. H. Wuryastuti, et al. "Effects of vitamin E on immune response of peripheral blood, colostrum and milk leukocytes." Journal of Animal Science 71 (1973): 2464-2472.

2. R. P. Tengerdy, et al." Vitamin E immunity and disease resistance." Diet and Resistance to Disease. M. Philips, and A. Baetz, eds. New York: Plenum Press, 1981.

3. K. V. Knowdley, et al. "Vitamin E deficiency and impaired cellular immunity related to intestinal fat malabsorption." Gastroenterology 102 (1992): 2139-2142.

4. K. Schmidt. "Interactions of antioxidative micronutrients with host defense mechanisms." A critical review. International Journal of Vitamin Nutrition Research 67 (1997): 307-311.

5. R. H. Prabhala, et al. "The effects of beta-carotene on cellular immunity in humans". Cancer 67 (1991): 1556-1560.

6. H. S. Garewal, et al. "Response of oral leukaplakia to beta-carotene." Journal of Clinical Oncology 8 (1990): 1715-1720.

7. R. Anderson, et al. "Ascorbate and cysteine mediated selective neutralisation of extracellular oxidants during N-formyl peptide activation of human phagocytes." Agents and Actions 20 (1987): 77-83.

8. C. S. Johnston, et al. "The effect of vitamin C nurture on compliment component Clq concentration in guinea pig plasma." Journal of Nutrition 117 (1987): 764-768.

9. S. Iwata, et al. "Thiol-mediated redox regulation of lymphocyte proliferation". Journal of Immunology 152 (1994): 5633-5642.

10. Roderer M, et al. "N-acetylcysteine inhibits latent HIV expression chronically infected cells." AIDS Research and Human Retroviruses 7 (1991): 563-567.

11. J. D. Bogden, et al. "Zinc and immunocompetence in the elderly: Base line data on zinc nutriture and immunity in unsupplemented subjects." American Journal of Clinical Nutrition 46 (1987): 101-109.

12. M. Dardenne, et al. "Contribution of zinc and other metals to the biological activity of serum thymic factor." Proceedings of the National Academy of Sciences 79 (1982): 5370-5373.

13. G. A. Ebeby, et al. "Reduction in duration of common colds by zinc gluconate lozenges in a double-blind study." Antimicrobial Agents and Chemotherapy 25 (1984) 25:20-24.

14. N. Boukaiba, et al. "A physicologial amount of zinc supplementation: Effects of nutritional, lipid, thymic status in an elderly population." American Journal of Clinical Nutrition 57 (1993): 566-572.

15. K. Folkers, et al. "Increase in levels of IgG in serum of patients treated with Coenzyme Q10." Research Communications in Molecular Pathology and Pharmacology 38 (1982): 335.

16. R. K. Chandra. "Effect of vitamin and trace element supplementation on immune responses and infection in the elderly subjects." Lancet 340 (1992): 1124-1127.

Chapter 10

1. R. Klein, et al. "Visual impairment and diabetes." Ophthalmology 91 (1984): 1-9.

2. U.S. Renal data system. "U.S. RDS 1994 annual data report". National Institute of Health, National Institute of Diabetes and Digestive and Kidney Diseases, Bethesda, Maryland, July 1994.

3. M. N. Diaz, et al. "Antioxidants and atherosclerotic heart disease". New England Journal of Medicine 337, no. 6 (August 7, 1997): 408-416.

4. J. R. Margolis, et al. "Clinical features of unrecognized myocardial infarction: Silent and symptomatic. Eighteen-year follow-up: The Framingham Study." American Journal of Cardiology 32 (1973): 1-7.

5. S. Vijayalingam, et al. "Abnormal antioxidant status in impaired glucose tolerance in non-insulin dependent diabetes mellitus." Diabetic Medicine 13, no. 8 (August 1996): 175-179.

6. I. A. Rud'ko, et al. "The results of a comparative study of the lipid perioxidation process and of the malondialdehyde level of the blood cells in patients with diabetic angiopathies and during insulin therapy." Terapeuticheskii Arkhiv 66, no. 10 (1994): 27-29.

7. P. A. Low, et al. "The role of oxidative stress and antioxidant treatment in experimental diabetic neuropathy." Diabetes 46 (September 1997 [supplement II]): S38-S42.

8. R. A. Anderson, and A. Kozlovsky. "Chromium intake, absorption, and excretion of subjects consuming self-selected diets." American Journal of Clinical Nutrition 41 (1985): 1177-1183.

9. E. Offenbacher, et al. "Beneficial effect of chromium-rich yeast on glucose tolerance and blood lipids in elderly subjects." Diabetes 29 (1980): 919-925.

10. G. Paolisso, et al. "Pharmacologic doses of vitamin E improve insulin action in healthy subjects and non-insulin dependent diabetic patients." American Journal of Clinical Nutrition 57 (1993): 650-656.

11. J. T. Salonen, et al. "Increased risk of non-insulin dependent diabetes mellitus at low plasma vitamin E concentrations: A four-year follow-up study in men." British Medical Journal 311 (1995): 1124-1127.

12. Z. T. Bloomgarden. "American Diabetes Association scientific sessions 1995: Magnesium deficiency, atherosclerosis, and health care." Diabetes Care 18 (1995): 1623-1627.

13. P. McNair, MD, et al. "Hypomagnesemia, a risk factor in diabetic retinopathy." Diabetes 27, no. 11 (November 1978): 1075-1077.

14. R. Whang. "Magnesium deficiency: Pathogenesis, prevalence, and clinical implications." American Journal of Medicine 82 (1987 [supplement IIIA]): 24-29.

Chapter 11

1.   R. R. Recker, et al. "Effect of estrogens and calcium carbonate on bone loss in post-menopausal women." Annals of Internal Medicine 87 (1977): 649-655.

2.   Y. Zhang, et al. "Bone mass and the risk of breast cancer among menopausal women." New England Journal of Medicine 336: no. 9 (February 27, 1997): 611-617.

3.   J. M. Burnell, et al. "The role of skeletal calcium deficiency in post-menopausal osteoporosis." Calcified Tissue Research 38 (1986): 187-192.

4.   B. Dawson-Hughes, MD, et al. "Effect of calcium and vitamin D supplementation on bone density in men and women 65 years of age or older." New England Journal of Medicine 337, no. 10 (September 4, 1997): 670-676.

5.   C. C. Johnston, Jr., MD, et al. "Calcium supplementation and increases in bone mineral density in children." New England Journal of Medicine 327, no. 2 (July 9, 1992): 82-87.

6.   B. M. Altura, and B. T. Altura. "Cardiovascular risk factors and magnesium: Relationships to atherosclerosis, ischemic heart disease and hypertension." Magnesium Trace Element 10 (1991-1992): 182-192.

7.   L. F. Barros, et al. "Magnesium treatment of acute myocardial infarction: Effects on necrosis in an occlusion/reperfusion dog model." International Journal of Cardiology 48 (1995): 3-9.

8.   G. E. Abraham, MD "The importance of magnesium in the management of primary post-menopausal osteoporosis." Journal of Nutritional Medicine 2 (1991): 165-178.

9.   P. M. Gallop, et al. "Carboxylated calcium-binding proteins and vitamin K." New England Journal of Medicine 302 (1980): 1460-1466.

10. J. P. Hart, et al. "Electrochemical detection of depressed circulating levels of vitamin K in osteoporosis." Journal of Clinical Endocrinology and Metabolism 60 (1985): 1268-1269.

11. A. Tomita. "Post-menopausal osteoporosis calcium study with vitamin K." Clinical Endocrinology (JPN) 19 (1971): 731-736.

12. J. C. Gallagher, et al. "Effective treatment with synthetic ones,25-dihydroxyvitamin D in post menopausal osteoporosis." Clinical Research 27 (1979): 366A.

13. R. N. Leach, Jr., and A. M. Muenster. "Studies on the role of manganese on bone formation." Journal of Nutrition 78 (1962): 51-56.

14. J. Raloff. "Reasons for boning up on manganese." Science News (September 27, 1986):199.. A. J. Grieco. Homocystinura: Pathogenetic mechanisms. American Journal of the Medical Sciences 273 (1977): 120-132.

16. F. H. Nielsen. "Boron-an overlooked element of potential nutritional importance." Nutrition Today (January/February 1988): 4-7.

17. F. H. Nielsen, C. D. Hunt, et al. "Effect of dietary boron on mineral, estrogen and testosterone metabolism in post-menopausal women." Faseb Journal 1 (1987): 394-397.

18. E. M. Carlisle "Silicone localization and calcification in developing bone." Federation Proceedings 28 (1969): 374.

19. O. S. Atik. "Zinc and senile osteoporosis." Journal of the American Geriatrics Society 31 (1983): 790-791.

BIONUTRITION

Chapter 13

1. National Research Council. "Recommended dietary allowances." 9th Edition Washington, D.C: National Academy of Press, 1980.
2. K.A. Muñoz, et al. "Food intake of United States children and adolescents compared with recommendation." Pediatrics 100: no. 3 (September 1997): 323-329.
3. G. Block. "Dietary guidelines and the results of food surveys." American Journal of Clinical Nutrition 53 (1991): 3565-75.
4. R. Beach. "Senate Document 264." 74th Congress, Second Session, June 1936.
5. F. E. Bear, S. J. Toth, and A. L. Prince. "Variation in mineral composition of vegetables." Soil Science Society Proceedings 13 (1948): 380.

Chapter 14

1. D. E. Hatoff, et al. "Hypervitaminosis A unmasked by acute viral hepatitis". Gastroenterology 82 (1982): 124-128.
2. K. J. Rothman, et al. "Teratogenecity of high vitamin A intake." New England Journal of Medicine 333 (1995): 1369-1373.
3. N. I. Krinsky, "Antioxidant function of carotenoids". Free Radical Biology and Medicine 7 (1989): 627-635.
4. R. D. Semba. "Vitamin A, immunity, and infection." Clinical Infectious Diseases 19 (1994): 489-499.
5. M. Murakoshi, et al. "Potent preventative action of alpha-carotene against carcinogenesis." Cancer Research 52 (1992): 6583-6587.
6. H. Gerster. "Anticarcinogenic effect of common carotenoids." International Journal of Vitamin and Nutrition Research 63 (1993): 93-212.
7. C. H. Hennekens. "Antioxidants and heart disease: epidemiology and clinical evidence." Clinical Cardiology 16 (1993 [supplement I]): 10-15.
8. J. M. Seddon, et al. "Dietary carotenoids, vitamins A, C, and E, and advanced age-related macular degeneration." JAMA 272, no. 18 (November 9, 1994): 1413-1420.
9. J. T. Landrum, et al. "A one-year study of the macular pigment: The effect of 140 days of a lutein supplement." Experimental Eye Research 65, no. 1 (July 1997): 57-62.
10. D. L. Morris, Ph.D., MD, et al. "Serum carotenoids and coronary artery disease." JAMA 272, no 18 (November 9, 1994): 1439-1441.
11. H.A.P. Pols, et al. "Vitamin D: A modulator of cell proliferation and differentiation." Journal of Steroid Biochemistry and Molecular Biology 37 (1990): 873-876.
12. M. N. Diaz, MD, et al. "Antioxidants and atheroscleroitic heart disease". New England Journal of Medicine 337, no. 6 (August 7, 1997): 408-416.
13. G. Paolisso, et al. "Pharmacologic doses of vitamin E improves insulin action in healthy subjects and non-insulin-dependent diabetic patients." American Journal of Clinical Nutrition 57 (1993): 650-656.
14. P. Kenkt, et al. "Vitamin E and cancer prevention." American Journal of Clinical Nutrition 53 (1991 [supplement I]): 283S-286S.
15. M. Steiner, MD, Ph.D., "Vitamin E: More than an antioxidant." Clinical Cardiology 16 (1993 [supplement I]): I16-I18.
16. K. Schmidt. "Interaction of antioxidative micronutrients with host defense mechanisms, a critical review." Internat J Vit Nutr Res 1997;67:307-311.
17. G. E. Hatch. "Asthma, inhaled oxidants, and dietary antioxidants." American Journal of Clinical Nutrition 61 (1995 [supplement]): 625S-630S.
18. I. Jialal, and S. Grundy. "Preservation of the endogenous antioxidants in low-density lipoprotein by ascorbate but not probucol during oxidative modification." Journal of Clinical Investigation 87 (1991): 597-601.
19. J. Simon. "Vitamin C and cardiovascular disease: A review." Journal of the American College of Nutrition 11 (1992): 107-125.

20. G. Block. "Vitamin C and cancer prevention: The epidemiologic evidence." American Journal of Clinical Nutrition 53 (1991): 270S-282S.

21. P. Knekt, et al. "Serum antioxidant vitamins and risk of cataract." British Medical Journal 305 (December 5, 1992): 1392-1394.

22. A. M. Vanderhagen, et al. "Free radicals and antioxidant supplementation: A review of their roles in age-related macular degeneration." Journal of the Amerian Optometry Association 64 (1993): 871-878.

23. C. Hunt, et al. "The clinical effects of vitamin C supplementation in elderly hospitalized patients with acute respiratory infections." International Journal of Vitamin and Nutrition Research 64 (1994): 212-219.

24. K. J. Meador, et al. "Evidence for the central cholinergic effect of high-dose thiamine." American Neurology 34 (1993): 724-726.

25. K. Meador. "Preliminary findings of high-dose thiamine in dementia of Alzheimer's type." American Journal of Geriatric Psychiatry and Neurology 6 (1993): 222-229.

26. D. R. Illingworth, et al. "Comparative effects of lovastatin and niacin in primary hypercholesterolemia." Archives of Internal Medicine 154 (1994): 1586-1595.

27. R.D. Reynolds, and C. L. Natta. "Depressed plasma pyredoxal-5-phosphate concentrations in adult asthmatics." American Journal of Clinical Nutrition 41 (1985): 684-688.

28. F. J. Kok, et al. "Low vitamin B-6 status in patients with acute myocardial infarction." American Journal of Cardiology 63 (1989): 513-516.

29. K. Folkers, and J. Ellis. "Successful therapy with vitamin B-6 and vitamin B-12 and the carpal tunnel syndrome and the need for determination of the RDA's for vitamin B-6 and B-2 disease states." Annals of the New York Academy of Sciences 585 (1990): 295-301.

30. C. Russ, et al. "Vitamin B-6 status of depressed and obsessive-compulsive patients." Nutr Rep Intl 27 (1983): 867-873.

31. C. L. Jones, and V. Gonzalez. "Pyridoxine deficiency: A new factor in diabetic neuropathy." Journal of the American Podiatry Association 68 (1978): 646-653.

32. E. Prein, and S. Gershoff. "Magnesium oxide-pyridoxine therapy for recurrent calcium oxalate calculi." Journal of Urology 112 (1974): 509-512.

33. M. K. Berman, et al. "Vitamin B-6 and premenstrual syndrome." Journal of American Dietic Association 90 (1990): 859-861.

34. J. B. Ubbink, et al. "Vitamin B-12, vitamin B-6 and folate nutritional status in men with hyperhomocysteine-mia." American Journal of Clinical Nutrition 57 (1993): 47-53.

35. VanGoor, et al. "Review, cobalamin deficiency and mental impairment in elderly people." Age and Aging 24 (1995): 536-542.

36. F. Abalan, et al. "Frequency of deficiencies of vitamin B-12 and folic acid in patients submitted to a geriatric-psychiatry unit." Encephale 10 (1984): 9-12.

37. Moghadasian, McManus, and Frohlich. "Homocysteine and coronary artery disease." Archives of Internal Medicine 157 (November 10, 1997): 2299-2305.

38. N. M. Werler, et al. "Periconceptional folic acid exposure and risk of occurrent neural tube defects." JAMA 269 (1993): 1257-1261.

39. L. E. Brattstrom, et al. "Folic acid responsive post menopausal homocysteinemia." Metabolism 34 (1985): 1073-1077.

40. N. Whitehead, et al. "Megaloblastic changes in the cervical epithelium association with oral contraceptive therapy and reversal with folic acid." JAMA 226 (1973): 1421-1424.

41. M. Botez, et al. "Effect of folic acid and vitamin B-12 deficiencies on 5-hytroxyindoleacetic acid in human cerebrospinal fluid." Annals of Neurology 12 (1982): 479-484.

42. G. Rosenberg, and K. L. Davis. "The use of cholinergic precursors in neuropsychiatric diseases." American Journal of Clinical Nutrition 36 (1982): 709-720.

BIONUTRITION

43. G. P. Littarru. "Energy and defense facts and prespectives on Coenzyme Q10 in biology and medicine." Casa Editrice Scientifica Intrenazionale (1994): 1-91.

44. K. Folkers, et al. "Biochemical rationale and myocardial tissue data on the effective therapy of cardiomyopathy with Coenzyme Q10." Proceedings of the American Academy of Science USA 282, no. 3 (1985): 901-904.

45. K. Folkers, et al. "Increase in levels of IGG in serum of patients treated with Coenzyme Q10". Research Communications in Chemical Pathology and Pharmacology 38 (1982): 35.

46. K. Lockwood, et al. "Progress on therapy of breast cancer with vitamin Q10 and the regression of metastasis." Biochemical and Biophysical Research Communications 212, no. 1 (July 6, 1995): 172-177.

47. T. Oda, and K. Hamamoto. "Effect of Coenzyme Q10 on the stress-induced decrease of cardiac performance in pediatric patients mitral valve prolapse." Jap Circ J 48 (1984): 1387.

48. T. Kamikawa, et al. "Effects of Coenzyme Q10 on exercise tolerance in chronic stable angina pectoris." American Journal of Cardiology 56 (1985): 247.

49. K. Fulers, and R. Simonsen. "Two successful double-blind trials with Coenzyme Q10 on muscular dystrophies and neurogenic atrophies." Biochemical and Biophysical Acta 1271 (1995): 281-286.

50. A. Reddi, et al. "Biotin supplementation improves glucose and insulin tolerances in genetically diabetic KK mice". Life Sciences 42 (1988): 1323-1330.

51. J. C. Coggeshall, et al. "Biotin status in plasma glucose in diabetics." Annals of the New York Academy of Sciences 447 (1985): 389-392.

52. A. Meister. "Selective modification of glutathione metabolism." Science 220 (1983): 472-477.

53. D. Bagchi, et al. "Oxygen free radical scavenging abilities of vitamins C and vitamin E, and a grape seed proanthocyanidin extract in vitro." Research Communication in Molecular Pathology and Pharmacology 1997 Feb; 95(2): 179-189.

54. R.M. Facino, et al. "Free radicals scavenging action and anti-enzyme activities of procyanidines from vitis vinifera." Arzneimittel-Forschung Drug Research 1994; 44(1), 5: 592-601.

Chapter 15

1. R. Recker. "Calcium absorption and achlorhydria." New England Journal of Medicine 313 (1985): 70-73.

2. J. R. Sowers, et al. "Calcium and hypertension." Journal of Laboratory and Clinical Medicine 114 (Year???):338-348.

3. J. R. Purvis, and A. Movahed. "Magnesium disorders and cardiovascular disease." Clinical Cardiology 15 (1992): 556-568.

4. E. M. Hampton, et al. "Intravenous magnesium therapy in acute myocardial infarction." Annals of Pharmacotherapy 28 (1994): 212-219.

5. R. M. McLean. "Magnesium and its therapeutic uses: A review." Am J Med 96 (1994): 63-76.

6. E. M. Skobeloff, et al. "Intravenous magnesium sulfate for the treatment of acute asthma in the emergency department." JAMA 262 (1989): 1210-1213.

7. T. Motoyama, et al. "Oral magnesium supplementation in patients with essential hypertension." Hypertension 13 (1989): 227-232.

8. J. S. Fernandes, et al. "Therapeutic effect of a magnesium salt in patients suffering from a mitro valvular prolapse and latent tetany." Magnesium 4 (1985): 283-289.

9. J. R. White, and R. K. Campbel. "Magnesium and diabetes: A review." Annals of Pharmacotherapy 27 (1993): 775-780.

10. N. M. Ramadan, et al. "Low brain magnesium and migraine." Headache 29 (1989): 590-593.

11. L. Cohen, and R. Kitzes. "Infared spectroscopy and magnesium content of bone mineral in osteoporotic women." Israel Journal of Medical Sciences 17 (1981): 1123-1125.

12. L. Spatling, and G. Spatling. "Magnesium supplementation in pregnancy a double-blind study." British Journal of Obstetrics and Gynecology 95 (1988): 120-125.

13. J. W. Piesse. "Nutritional factors in the premenstrual syndrome." International Clinical Nutrition Review 4 (1994): 54-81.

14. N. Boukaiba, et al. "A physiological amount of zinc supplementation: Effects on nutritional, lipid, and thymic status in the elderly population." American Journal of Clinical Nutrition 57 (1993): 566-572.

15. A. Netter, et al. "Effect of zinc administration on plasma testosterone, dihydrotestosterone and sperm count." Archives of Andrology 7 (1991): 69-73.

16. D. A. Newsome, et al. "Oral zinc and macular degeneration." Archives of Ophthalmology 106 (1988): 192-198.

17. J. Constantinidis. "Treatment of Alzheimer's Disease by zinc compounds." Developmental Research 27 (1992): 1-14.

18. F. H. Neilsen. "Effect of dietary boron on mineral, estrogen, and testosterone metabolism in postmenopausal women." FASEB Journal 1 (1987): 394-397.

19. W. Mertz. "Chromium in human nutrition: A review." Journal of Nutrition 123, no. 6 (1993): 626-633.

20. L. C. Clark, et al. "Effects of selenium supplementation for cancer prevention in patients with carcinoma of the skin." JAMA 276, no. 24 (1996): 1957-1963.

21. M. Roy. "Supplementation with selenium in human immune cell function." Biological Trace Element Research 41 (1994): 103-114.

22. F. J. Kok, et al. "Decreased selenium levels in acute myocardial infarction." JAMA 261 (1989): 1161-1164.

23. E. Munthe, and J. Aseth. "Treatment of rheumatoid arthritis with selenium and vitamin E." Scandinavian Journal of Rheumatology 53 (1984 [supplement]):103.

24. S. Karakucuk, et al. "Selenium concentrations serum, lens, aqueous humor of patients with senile cataracts." Archives of Optholmology Scandinavia 73 (1995): 329-332.

25. J. T. Salonen, et al. "High stored iron levels are associated with excess risk of myocardial infarction in eastern Finnish men." Circulation 86 (1992): 803-811.

Chapter 16

1. D. E. Hatoff, et al. "Hypervitaminosis unmasked by acute viral hepatitis." Gastroenterology 82 (1982): 124-128.

2. R. Olson, ed. Nutrition Reviews: Present Knowledge of Nutrition, 6th ed. Washington, DC: Nutrition Foundation, 1989, pp. 96-107.

3. K. J. Rothman, et al. "Teratogenecity of high vitamin A intake." New England Journal of Medicine 333 (1995): 1369-1373.

4. Alpha-tocopherol, beta-carotene cancer prevention study group. "The effect of vitamin E and beta-carotene on incidence of lung cancer and other cancers in male smokers." New England Journal of Medicine 330 (1994): 1029-1035.

5. M. Steiner , MD, Ph.D. "Vitamin E: More than an antioxidant." Clinical Cardiology 16 (1993 [supplement I]): I-16-I-18.

6. M. S. Seelig. "Magnesium deficiency with phosphate and vitamin D excess: Roland pediatric cardiovascular nutrition." Cardiovascular Medicine 3 (1978): 637-650.

7. J. M. McKenney, et al. "A comparison of the efficacy and toxic effects of sustained-versus immediate-release niacin in hypercholesterolemic patients." JAMA 271 (1994): 672-677.

8. G. J. Parry, and D. E. Bredesen. "Sensory neoropathy with low-dose pyridoxine." Neurology 35 (1985): 1466-1468.

9. A. N. Fan, and K. W. Kizer. "Selenium: nutritional, toxicological and clinical aspects." Western Journal of Medicine 153 (1990): 160-167.

Subject Index

BIONUTRITION

BIONUTRITION